Facing Death Together

The Story of Our Losing Battle with Cancer

Jordan B. Smith Jr. Ed.D.

Kindle Press

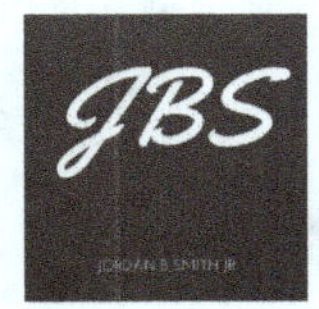

Contents

Introduction

This book is a personal memoir of a very traumatic life experience, which lasted 15 months. It was a very stressful time for me, which ended in the death of my wife, Joyce Ann Smith. I loved her dearly. This is a true story of how we faced death together, after receiving a diagnosis that she had stage 4 inoperable lung cancer. It took us over four months for her doctors to finally make that diagnosis. Joyce had been a lifetime smoker since she was 16 years old. In 2013 her doctors told her to stop smoking or else the cancerous tissue would likely return. After we both stopped smoking, we were still being exposed to second-hand smoke, while vacationing to many casinos, in Nevada for over 6 years. I remember watching TV commercials of an old man, who was dying from cancer, speaking through a voice box in his throat, and many other commercials against the dangers of smoking. I thought at the time this was never going to happen to us.

Cigarette sales are still on the shelves today, even though local governments in California have taxed them severely. We were hooked on nicotine and the lifestyle of the vivid TV ads making smoking look cool. We ignored the warnings for far too many years. Cancer is not a joke. It is not a hoax! I have learned to heed the health warnings of medical doctors and scientist.

Many Americans need to understand that politics can never defeat a pandemic. When I am sick, I don't go to see an airline pilot, a soldier, a governor, or a mayor of a city. I go to a qualified licensed medical professional. When I started working as a teacher, our health provider did a full physical in 2003, and advised both of us to stop smoking. We continued to smoke. Each year, during our annual physical, for the next ten years we did not heed the doctor's recommendations, until the doctor told Joyce that she would get cancer once again and might die if she didn't stop. I am fortunate enough to still be alive to write this book and to say these words in order to save one life. There are members of our family, who still continue to smoke. Please, listen to your medical doctors. During this COVID-19 medical emergency I advise everyone to follow the guidance of your local medical professionals. There is no immunity against cancer, while smoking cigarettes. Likewise, COVID-19 is real and at the time of publication of this book there have been 188,000+ deaths and 6.2+ million cases in America since March 2020.

During her third month of chemotherapy, Joyce asked me to begin writing about our experience, while facing death together, so people would become aware of what to expect from their medical providers, insurance companies, and funeral homes. I am thankful that she had the opportunity to pass while she was at home, surrounded by her loving family. Those Americans, who have died from the Coronavirus pandemic, as of July 2020, were not lucky enough to have friends or family members in attendance at their funeral or memorial services. The COVID-19 pandemic is surging in America as I write this today, and the virus is being spread by many young people who think they are invincible. Those who do not know history are destined to repeat the mistakes of the past.

There are many things about insurance claims and obtaining services from your medical providers, I wish I had understood. We had prepared our wills and made a Living Trust, in the event one of us died. No one prepares you for the events prior to a diagnosis of cancer. When a doctor gives you 12-18 months to live you have no idea of the hell you and your family are about to embark on. Those 15 months felt like an eternity in hell. It was a bad dream you wished you could wake up from but could not open your eyes.

Joyce lost 65 pounds due to her illness and I lost 23 pounds due to the stress of trying to balance my work and take care of her. Her dying wish was for me to complete this book, so that others might be better prepared to handle a terminal illness. The scheduled release date for this book will coincide with her birthday on August 6, 2020 which would have been her 74th birthday. The profits from this book will help in the research for cancer, and contribute to the funding of educational scholarships for students in need.

Preface

Hopefully, this book will help eliminate any unnecessary pain, and confusion when dealing with a life changing terminal illness. Cancer is as real as this COVID-19. People don't realize the lasting effects of a major illness. Once cancer is in your body it doesn't go away. The major mistake of medical professionals and the Trump administration's handling of the pandemic, in 2020 was releasing data and findings, without explanations of its' concepts. Most people in America lack the conceptual understanding and knowledge of exponential functions. The first wave of the coronavirus pandemic never ended and got much worse because of the lack of a national policy and failed leadership of the Trump administration. A lot of young people who did not die are experiencing long term damage to their body that will not surface until years later. The same is for the long term harmful internal damage of smoking cigarettes throughout one's lifetime.

Prologue

I first met Joyce in December of 2002 while I was working as a Karaoke DJ, at a local hotspot night club called the Main Event, in San Jacinto, CA. She came into the night club to attend a meeting to discuss the arrangements for her daughter, Christina's wedding, scheduled for June 2003. At the time I thought Joyce was still married, because Christina (Christy) had also introduced me to her father earlier that evening, who was also at the club to attend the meeting. A few months later, in February 2003, I transitioned to work as a bartender on the weekends, working with Christina. I still hosted the Karaoke show on Thursday nights. One of those weekday nights Christina had encouraged her mother to get out of the house and find a new life or have a life. I was setting up and testing my karaoke system when I noticed Christina enter the bar with her mom. When they arrived, Christina gave her mom a Corona with lime and salt around the rim. I left the stage, and came to the bar to say hello, and I asked Christy to fix me a drink. Christy re-introduced me to her Mom (Joyce). I remembered seeing Gary, her husband, and inquired about him. Joyce told me, "Well he is back home in northern California. We have been divorced for over 20+ years." She went on to explain how she had been alone and single for many years and the only reason for her being here tonight was because Christy had bugged the heck out of her. I went back to start hosting karaoke and later Christy asked me to sing a song to her mother. I asked her what song and she said, "get her in the right mood, sing I'll Make Love to You." I had no idea the effect that love song would have on Joyce. I sang that song up close and personal, as I had done many times before. She had a smile on her face and was having a good time sitting at the bar drinking and smoking with Christy's bar customers. She really enjoyed herself. I asked Joyce, before she left, whether or not she had fun tonight. She said, "Yes, I did. I think I'll come back again. Hopefully, I will see you again." She placed her hand out to shake mine and said "goodnight."

Joyce came back the next night with a mission. That mission was to get me. Little did I know I was going to be her Valentine gift. Somehow, later that night, I asked her what she wanted for Valentine's Day and she said without hesitation, "I want you.". I asked her, "Well, what about Christy? She replied, "it's my house not hers." Joyce took me home with her that night. When she opened the door, she said, "Now remember this mess is not mine." Little did she know that she was about to get involved with a United States Marine. Cleaning house was not a problem! I remember saying that I just wanted to cuddle and go to sleep. Joyce had other ideas as she started to cuddle up to me.

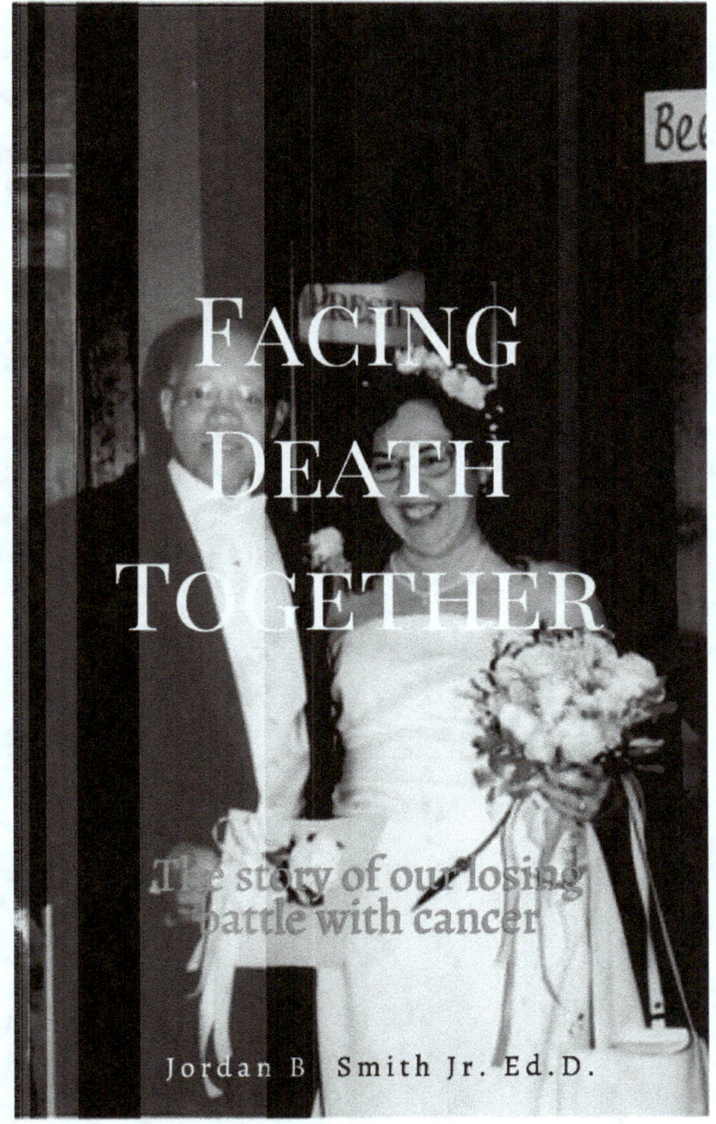
FACING
DEATH
TOGETHER
The story of our losing
battle with cancer
Jordan B. Smith Jr. Ed.D.

Chapter 1 - Spring Break

It was the first day of my vacation, during the first week in April 2018, and I was on spring break while working as a public-school teacher. I was ready for a long-needed break,from working long hours, during the present school year. We always looked forward to our vacations. Since being married in 2003, we had taken at least one vacation each year. Each trip was in celebration of another year together and working hard to make our dreams come true.

I was always busy with my work as a teacher, working 60 plus hours a week. I began my teaching career at the age of 50, after serving my last days as a Marine Logistics Officer. In the spring of 2018, everything at work was at its peak performance, with more recognition, and awards clearly in my future. I loved my job as a schoolteacher,as I was able to help students to overcome past problems in their life and to somehow "straighten the rudder," and turn their lives around.

For me it was always about math and critical thinking, but the only reason I could do these things was because of the love and support of my wife, Joyce. She was the foundation of our family. Most importantly, Joyce was my best friend and confidant. We both had many failed relationships and marriages, prior to getting together as a couple, our marriage in September 2003 was a match made in heaven.

We were best friends, lovers, Mr. & Mrs. Santa Claus, and living happily together. In the spring of 2018, we were planning for our future retirement together for the rest of our lives. I had just turned 64 years old and Joyce would have been 72 years old, on her upcoming birthday, in August. On her birthday we would have been married nearly 16 years.

Our marriage brought together her daughter and son, with my three sons. These two different families were merged into one cohesive loving family. During the past 15 years, we planned for nearly everything, except for the events about to happen on our upcoming vacation. Spring breaks for the past six years had been planned out well in advance, including the finite details of how to hold and keep most of our vacation money, from the Treasure Island Casino. We enjoyed being together away from work and family. Although Joyce had been retired for nearly three years, her daily life was consumed with adult children, who were still struggling to *get a foot in the door*, of responsible living. We would routinely turn off our cell phones and not answer any family calls during our vacations. We posted pictures on Facebook and sent daily text messages to keep family aware of our locations, and travel plans. I was not considering retirement, as I enjoyed my work and the income, which provided a comfortable lifestyle.

During our first few years of taking our vacations to casinos, we would spend everything we had saved for the vacation. The result was the casino received 100% of our money. A stroke of good luck came on our vacation trip in 2010, when the Pala cashier shared her strategy of always taking money home. She would use five-dollar bills to play on a slot machine, and whenever the machine hit, she would immediately cash out and save the ticket. We learned a valuable lesson to never put these winning tickets back into a slot machine. We saved them until the day of our departure. From that moment on, we would always leave our casino vacations with money in our pockets. During the past 9 years we brought home 87% of what we put into the machines. This strategy made every vacation trip more enjoyable for both of us. Our trip back home always included a stop at our credit union, to make a deposit into our savings account, as a nest egg for our next vacation trip.

Our friends for the past 15 years, Barbara and Jim had always spent time in Laughlin, because their rooms were always compensated, by the casino. They shared with us the secret was to always spend your money at one hotel and then that casino would invite you back and give you free rooms. So, we followed their lead and now we were offered free rooms each year in Las Vegas and Laughlin. Most of the time we upgraded our room, because of the discount offered us by the casino. As a result, for the past three years, we have always enjoyed spacious luxury suites.

Our trip during the first week of April, 2018, was in the Tower Suite, at Treasure Island, on the Las Vegas strip. Our room was a luxurious 900+ square foot suite, with two bathrooms and a jacuzzi bathtub, which overlooked the strip, and a mountain view.

The road trip from home to Vegas was about four and a half hours. Everything seemed to be perfect, but something was wrong, and I had no idea what was about to happen, in the next few months Something was about to change our life together forever. Sadly, Joyce had been keeping a secret from me, as she did not want me to over-react and cancel our vacation plans.

The difficult part about going on vacation was leaving our home and our loving pet, Tommie who was a cute little dog, with a big personality. Joyce's sister (Lynn) would house sit and take care of

"Tommie" whenever we went on vacation. "Tommie boy" loved the company of Lynn's dog Whitney. Tommie boy was being spoiled because for the past four years, he did not have to go to the kennel. Lynn always came to stay while we traveled. It worked out great for all concerned.

After six years of annual vacations we would always pack-up and take way too much stuff. Together we were like scouts always wanting to be prepared.

Many years ago, my first cousin shared with me a secret for receiving excellent service. He stated that wealthy people believed that tipping was a way to guarantee good service. They know, "To Insure Prompt Service (TIPS)" should be paid in advance, not after the service had been performed. Over the years of vacationing this has proven to be true time and time again. Our vacations were all about, finally spending time together as a couple, and putting behind all the drama regarding our grown children, back at home.

Room service was an absolute must for Joyce. She loved room service and the smell of coffee and other foods she did not have to cook. We went out to dinner every night choosing different restaurants, without thinking about the price, as we had saved enough money to enjoy these vacations together.

Unknown to us at that time, we would soon be spending even more time together, but not for the reasons both of us would have thought possible. Joyce (Ms. Claus) had already purchased presents for our annual Christmas Eve party. Every year, I would tell my co-workers and friends, that I had married Mrs. Claus. Many of our co-workers and friends would follow her lead in preparing for Christmas each year. My male friends would simply laugh, and female co-workers would be astounded that her shopping list would be complete before Halloween. I had finally found and married the right woman. Even on vacation Joyce would update her calendar ensuring that everyone in our family would receive a gift, on their birthday and Christmas. Joyce was not just about Christmas, but every birthday and special event.

No matter what the circumstances Joyce always hid a gift, which would bring happiness to other people. I tried as much as possible to make her happy by bringing her small gifts and flowers, at unexpected times and even tickling her, for a brief moment, even though she hated it.

It was a beautiful California sunny day, scattered clouds in the distance, 85 degrees, and clear blue skies above. Everything was perfect for this trip to Treasure Island, in Vegas, on April Fool's Day in 2018. After many days of preparation our car was packed to the brim with snacks and all the necessities for our trip. We pulled out of the driveway in our 55+ community, and began our trip to the Vegas strip.

Chapter 2 – On the Road Again-
Another Trip to Vegas

We had the driving routine, on long trips, down to a science. We would normally take turns driving, with me driving the first couple of hours and then Joyce would take over driving for two hours. I would then drive the final hours to the hotel. However, during our last two trips I had to take over the total driving duties. I did not think anything about it at the time.

We kept a cooler behind the passenger's seat filled with snacks and drinks. Our favorites were cashews, sunflower seeds, and caffeine filled cokes which kept us awake. Joyce enjoyed being the co-pilot and snack server, as we embarked on our trips to Vegas. She also loved our brief stops in Baker or Barstow, for a sit-down fast food meal.

When Joyce and I met I was a Disc Jockey (DJ)/Karaoke entertainer. My music tastes ran closer to R&B old school genre of soul music. Joyce loved Def Leppard, The Eagles, Ricky Nelson, Neil Diamond, and Rod Stewart, to name a few. I enjoyed Earth, Wind, & Fire; Marvin Gaye, Barry White and Lionel Richie. We decided that country music would be our choice of music, on the road, as we both enjoyed this type of music together.

Since I had taken over the driving, country music kept me awake and sharp, while driving to Vegas and on our long trips to San Antonio, Texas to visit my two sons. We would share the driving duties on our trips to San Antonio, with each of us driving three hours, before stopping at a hotel to spend the night. We no longer had the stamina to drive straight through for nine to ten hours a day.

On our last trip to Texas I did all of the driving, as Joyce began having some discomfort. Six months after that 2013 trip to Texas, Joyce was diagnosed with Vulva Cancer and was out of work due to her resulting surgery. Since that surgery, Joyce continued to have routine checkups every six months as suggested by her doctors. In 2017 her checkups were changed from bi-annual, to annual checkups. Since then, all of her tests showed negative results of any cancer tissue. This was great news for both of us.

We were so happy to hear she was cancer free at last. We began planning our retirement together. Afterall, Joyce was confident, because a palm reader (psychic) told her she would live to be 82 years old. Almost everything this physic told her had come true, thus far, which also included finding me as her soul mate and partner for the rest of her life. Little did I know at the time how true this was.

The physic told her she would meet the love of her life in her 50's and that her wedding would be so close to her daughters, that it could have been a double wedding. I was just another example of the physic reading coming true. Joyce was very happy. She was retired, living in a beautiful home, with a loving husband

and could fulfill her role as Ms. Claus, grandma, and now great grandma. The physic said that she would not die from cancer. So much for palm readers!

Joyce had beaten cancer once, and now being worry free, could enjoy our vacations once again, with the love of her life. However, something was wrong, and Joyce chose not to share this information with me, as she did not want to spoil our long-awaited vacation. Vacations were our way of leaving the drama at home behind us.

Joyce told her visiting sister, "I am so excited about our vacation to Treasure Island in Vegas. This trip has become an annual event for us during the past several years while I was on Spring Break." Unknown to me, at the time, Joyce was feeling some discomfort that she thought was under control. For the past15 years Joyce had a daily routine of drinking her morning coffee and having a bowel movement (BM) before going to work. It was automatic like clockwork. The morning we left on this trip she had difficulty having a BM. I later discovered that this would not be the first time.

Joyce laughingly says', "It's no big deal, I will go poop when we get to Vegas." However, she had no such luck during the next four days. We had booked the Tower Suits for five nights.

We normally liked to stop at a midpoint, normally at Barstow to stretch, eat, and use the facilities. I was slightly concerned and continued to ask Joyce if she needs to stop for a restroom break. "I'm ok, I will go when we get there, honey. Really, I'm ok. I'm a big girl", she says while looking out the car window. Joyce drifted off to sleep, as we cross the state line, and fell asleep as we pass by the Buffalo Bills Casino.

I adjusted the view on the navigation screen to check for my exit to the hotel. I looked to my right and noticed Joyce was sleeping. I maneuvered, correctly this time as the car hugged the ramp onto Spring Mountain Road. I pulled into the valet isle and nudge Joyce saying "We're here honey!" I stepped out of the car and stretched my arms over my head while yawning. While putting my Navy cap on, I helped Joyce out of the car.

After giving the bell captain a $20 tip, the porter gathered up our 13 pieces of luggage and belongings. We held hands and as we walked to the check-in desk, inside the hotel, using the invited guest isle. It was VIP treatment once again.

This was our first time staying in the Tower Suite at Treasure Island. Joyce loved the fact that it was close to the elevators. As we opened the large double door she just gasped, "This room is huge and bigger than the Venetian. She walked quickly to the largest of the two bathrooms, and said, "I think I got to go." She had chosen the bathroom with the vanity mirror and more counter space for her medicine and makeup. There was a large jacuzzi bathtub and a huge glass enclosed shower. I asked her, "Well, did you go?", while pausing to look at the number of jets in the tub. I turned to her and asked, "How long have you been constipated?" She responded, "three days I think." I was slightly upset that she had not shared this with me, until now. This was not unusual for Joyce to hide non harmful, physical discomforts. I watched as sheoyce took out her make-up bag, now full of prescription pill bottles. It normally took her about thirty minutes to separate all of her pills each week. Luckily, we had a good medical insurance program. If we did not have insurance, her medications would have cost over $1,000 a month.

Chapter 3 – The Bookkeeper – A Midwestern Tart

J oyce was retiring after 40 years as a business bookkeeper. I loved the fact that I had found a woman who could do taxes and handle the family finances. She was well organized and reconciled our bank accounts on a daily basis. During the last 15 years, we never had a late payment. Joyce was a strong independent woman and was quite stubborn at times, which was one of her loving characteristics. She reminded me of the woman, who portrayed the grandma, in the movie *Soul Food*. At 72 years of age, Joyce was looking forward to spending the final ten years of her life with her prince charming, which would fulfill the psychic's prophecy.

I quite often recalled the words of Peggy Wishmire (Joyce's Mom) during our first Christmas together. My new mother-in-law gave me some quick advice. Peggy pulled me aside to speak privately, while Joyce was busy in the kitchen, preparing food for our annual Christmas Eve family get together. Our first Christmas (2003) would be the last time Joyce would cook alone. Little did she know, but her time in the kitchen would dramatically change as I considered myself quite the chef.

Our first Christmas together, and in the coming years, would bring about the most wonderous times any family could have imagined. During preparation for our first Christmas Eve party, Peggy whispered to me, "You just keep making her smile young man." Peggy turned away then stopped and added, "If you don't, you'll be sorry you ever met me." Peggy held up her index and pinkie finger and said, "this is not what it seems, but this is for those who don't deserve this (holding up only the middle finger indicating FU)." I was in shock and just chuckled, with a smile and a wink saying, "Ms. Wishmire you are one of a kind and that's for sure. You're a country hoot!"

Peggy strongly stated, "You can make any decision you want, but you can never interfere with Christmas!" And with that she smoothly turned around, leaning slightly on her custom brown walking cane, with the golden handle, and left me standing alone in the master bedroom. As she walked out, I saw her wiping tears from the corner of her eyes. She walked back to the living room to enjoy time with the rest of the family. You could hear the sounds of laughter coming from the living room next to our beautiful eight-foot Christmas tree. It was the most beautiful tree, my two boys (John and Jared) had ever seen. It had so many presents under it that it took up half the space in our living room.

Peggy Wishmire was a sweet old mid-western tart of a woman. She was a no-nonsense type of lady and I came to understand over the years about compromise and bending over backwards to help family members, whenever they were in need. All of our children joined together as step siblings in our marriage. Some of these adult children were far from angels and during the 15+ years of our marriage they burdened us financially and emotionally.

Each year since 2004, I concentrated on increasing my income. Although I was a mathematician, I chose to have Joyce handle all of our finances, such as paying the bills and keeping the budget. Her bookkeeping experience made her ideal for this task. She loved doing this and it made her a happy wife.

Chapter 4 – There's No Place Like Home

We used our vacation time to recharge our batteries, before returning to face the challenging ups and downs of being parents, grandparents, and great-grandparents. During this vacation trip to Vegas, Joyce revealed that she had not had a bowel movement during the last four days. She then decided to take Magnesium Citrate, which gave her diarrhea, and she had to remain in our hotel room the entire third day of our vacation. I was very concerned, and asked her "Are you sure you're ok?" She told me "I'm ok. You go ahead and have some fun and make some more money for this year's Christmas."

As I went back down to the casino, I told her to call me if she needed me. I played for a couple more hours, but I could not keep my mind off of Joyce, while playing the slot machines. I started losing more than winning and then suddenly I hit a Jackpot. I thought to myself "it's time to cash out and go home." So, out of concern for her health, I decided to cancel the remainder of our trip, after only three nights. I wanted to return to home to California, in order to be closer to Joyce's doctor and hospital.

During our trip home I reflected on my experiences when my

mother died, prematurely, at the age of 45. My mom (Gladys) did not have a Will and very little insurance, when she passed away. I reminisced about how Joyce helped her mother create a Living Trust, which made it easier for us to complete her final wishes, prior to her death in 2008. Joyce and I decided to create a Revocable Living Trust, reviewing and updating it often, since its inception in 2017.

We kept and maintained life insurance policies on both of our lives to ensure that all our final expenses and wishes would be met. I believed you could never have enough insurance. I frequently stated, "I have no worries, as I am more than fully insured." Joyce jokingly responded, "Ok, Mr. smart ass!" "Yes, and I love you too, but I do have four college degrees to back up my smart ass!", I retorted back to her.

I have always been an over cautious defensive driver, and especially now on our trip back home to California. The last thing I wanted was for both of us to die in a car accident, as Joyce's son Greg had done in a horrible car accident on May 14, 2013. Greg's death still brings about past memories, and periods of depression for Joyce and her only daughter Christina. We had always been responsible parents, taking precautions to ensure our children would not be burdened financially, upon our death.

On this trip to Vegas, I took the back roads, in order to avoid Interstate 15, by taking Interstate 10 East to Amboy near the U. S. Marine Base in 29 Palms, California. But that route had several miles of no cell phone service, so on the return trip home I wanted to make sure we were within a reasonable distance to restroom facilities. On the way back home, we stopped in Barstow and arrived safely back home after a four-and-a-half-hour trip.

Upon arriving home, we are greeted by our dog Tommie who goes "nuts" as he waited by the door, listening for our entry keypad and the sounds of chimes on our alarm system, as the back door opens. He was so excited to see his mom and dad, back home once again. There's no place like home!

Although I was disappointed that our trip was cut short, I am now worried about Joyce and very tired from the long drive back home. As I lay down for a nap, before falling asleep, I thought, "Is this the first time Joyce has been constipated for this long?"

Chapter 5 – Something to Worry About?

Luckily, Joyce, had already scheduled a doctor's appointment prior to our return home. On April 9, 2018 Joyce's primary care doctor advised her to have a colonoscopy, which was overdue. She refused to go ignoring her doctor's advice, which would prove to be a drastic mistake. However, she did start to take stool softeners, with a mild laxative, during the remainder of April.

For the rest of April Joyce would suffer severe constipation for about three days, followed by diarrhea, after using either milk of magnesia, magnesium citrate, or Dulcolax. You name it and she did it, but unfortunately, with the same end results. She was having severe stomach cramps and back pain on a daily basis. Ibuprofen and Tylenol PM did not help her sleep throughout the night. In fact, she could not lay flat on her back or in bed for any length of time, without severe pain. Yes, something was terribly wrong.

I would wake up several times during the night to find Joyce sitting up in bed leaning forward sleeping. This was the only way she could get relief from her lower back pain. This pain was mostly due to her constipation. Joyce was not getting very much rest. I also spent many restless nights, becoming more and more concerned that this was not merely a case of constipation.

I would often reach across the bed during the night to check on her and awaken to find the other side of our bed was empty. I would often panic and jump out of bed calling her name, and would find her completely asleep on her throne of pain, the master bedroom toilet.

I would often wake up to find Joyce not in bed beside me. I would look out the opening in the window shutters and notice that it was still dark outside. "What the f%&&^7 time is it", I thought to myself as I turned to get out of bed. "Well I know it's not 5 AM, because Tommie is still sleeping", I whispered to myself.

I rubbed my eyes while reaching out my hand to the nightstand, in search of my glasses and checked the time on the clock. It was 2:30 AM and my alarm had not sounded. I wondered where Joyce was, so I got up to go to the bathroom, where I found Joyce once more sitting on her royal throne.

"Hey what are you doing, are you ok?", I asked her through the crack in the bathroom door. "Same old shit, just a brand-new day", Joyce said with a little grin and a chuckle. "Just another day in paradise", she continued. "I just wish everything would go back to normal. I've had a routine for the last 50 damn years. Life was simple. I would have my coffee with hazelnut creamer, two sugars, wait about 30 minutes and then another F-day in paradise and relief." Joyce continues, "Now I drink my coffee, and nothing works. I wait and wait and wait. When is this going to stop?"

Chapter 6 – The Unwanted Guest Returns

Cancer was no stranger to Joyce, she had experienced two different discoveries, in the past. The first time was when she was in her 30's and her pap smear came back abnormal. Upon further examination a spot was discovered on her uterus. The second discovery was in 2013 when her doctor found a spot on her vulva. Both times her surgeries were successful and her follow-up scans found no trace of the abnormal cancer tissue.

After her surgery, Joyce was required to undergo a physical examination and a tissue exam every six months, as a follow-up routine. At that time her doctor warned her if she did not stop smoking, her cancer would return. I didn't believe she could stop, but because of her love for me and her desire to have a long life together, we both decided to stop at the same time. When two people love each dearly, they will do anything to stay together. Neither of us considered the trips to Las Vegas and Laughlin, with all the second-hand smoke was a dangerous health concern. Boy, we were wrong! Second-hand smoke is extremely dangerous and should be avoided whenever possible. Everyone should listen to all the medical and scientific data, concerning health and lifestyle decisions.

Joyce had never had a computerized tomography (CT) scan, which would have discovered any abnormalities. Her doctors never thought of performing this procedure. I would find out later in the coming months that anyone with a long history of smoking was still at risk of getting cancer for up to ten years after quitting. A normal precautionary treatment is an annual CT scan. Routine examinations did not discover what was causing Joyce's constipation and stomach pains. We would make many more visits to doctors, before the right procedure would clearly identify what was at the root of her problem. What Joyce was experiencing, on a day to day basis, were symptoms of a much deeper problem.

Between April and the end of May 2018, every visit to the hospital (15 trips to Urgent Care and Emergency Room) provided the same recommendations to use fiber and laxatives, as solutions for constipation and stomach pains. The repeated x-ray's and ultrasound scans showed large pockets of gas in the intestines. The repeated answer was to drink more water, take stool softeners, eat more fiber, walk and take laxatives. Now Joyce also needed to also take gas-ex, after every meal. Although the advice was consistent, it was not enough to release the pain Joyce was experiencing, on a daily basis. We knew something else was wrong.

The constipation problems had lasted for over six weeks. I was always nagging Joyce to consume more water and to walk more often. She would not do this by herself. This task was going to be nearly impossible, because I had to return to work.

Since February of 2018, Joyce had been going for her annual

checkup with her favorite doctor. He was one of the doctors who performed her surgery in 2013. She was given a private number to contact him if there were any health concerns. During a telephone appointment with him in May 2018, she shared her frustrations with her continual constipation and pain. It was much later that I read the following clinical notes by Dr. Sherman:

______________________________________Beginning of notes

Patient contacted

For the last month+ she has been unable to have a normal BM

Using fiber and stool softeners.

Mag citrate on 2 occasions.

Straining a lot.

Denies prior issues like this

A/P

- f/u 5/25

- cool planned

- call or return to clinic sooner if problems arise

Dr. Sherman arranged to expedite the colonoscopy (May 22) with Dr June which came back with signs of

Colon polyp(s),

Hemorrhoids, internal

Diverticulosis

None of these findings could explain the continuous lower back pain and constipation. Dr. Sherman does a follow-up to the colonoscopy and records the following notes:

History:

Patient presents with:

CONSTIPATION: COLONOSCOPY F/UP

She complains of new onset constipation.

BMs only normal when taking Dulcolax. Otherwise BMs hard, difficult to evacuate. Took mag citrate when really bad. Not taking fiber supplement.

Also notes new left lower quadrant tenderness

BP 118/66 | Pulse 64 | Temp 99.6 °F (37.6 °C) (Tympanic) | Ht 1.626 m (5' 4") | Wt. 92.1 kg (203 lb.) | BMI 34.84 kg/m^2

Physical Exam

Abdominal:

Genitourinary:

Genitourinary Comments: DRE: no masses, very small rectocele

A/P

- start fiber supplement

- continue Dulcolax, wean off in 1-2 weeks if BMs improved on fiber

- improve PO fluids

- CT to r/o hernia

- if persists, consider MR def

____End of Notes

One day as Joyce was watching TV, she quickly got up and ran to the bathroom. I was preparing to start cooking on the grill, when I suddenly heard Joyce scream out, "Ow!" I ran into the house to the bathroom to find she had somehow injured her leg and could not get off the toilet. While trying to rise from the toilet, she had severely strained her leg, and could not walk without severe pain.

I told her I was going to get the car", she refused to go telling me, "No, I'm not going back to the damn urgent care", Joyce said while moaning slightly. "I'll be alright. I don't know what happened. How does someone hurt their leg getting off of the damn toilet? I guess I'm getting old", she laughingly said. I helped her up and noticed that she could barely walk without pain. I went to get her mother's walking cane for her and decided that this was not going to help. I then went to my favorite store (Amazon) and ordered a cane, a walker, and handicap toilet seats for both our bathrooms in anticipation of her future needs.

Chapter 7 - The Balancing Act - Old Farts - Living with Pain and Losing a Child

After all of the tests Joyce had been through, nothing seemed to alleviate her pain. We began to adjust to her new way of living, of being constipated for three days, with a magnesium flush on the fourth day. She simultaneously developed pain in her right leg, which required the daily use of her cane. She could no longer drive the car. This went on for about six weeks.

The month of, May 2018, was a difficult one for her, as this was the anniversary of the accidental death of her only son Greg who died on May 14, 2013. "I really miss him even though he would screw things up and always get caught", Joyce reflected about him, while sitting on her throne. "I can remember being at home and seeing money being withdrawn from my bank account. He was at the casino using my damn ATM card." Joyce continued, "I don't know why he does such things, because he always gets caught."

"I loved him even though he made bad decisions like stealing my car and only getting one block away from the house, because he flipped the finger at an undercover cop", Joyce continued while laughing with tears running down her face. "I loved that boy, but sometimes he was so stupid. He was always getting caught!"

God doesn't make much sense sometimes. "I think God needs to fire his secretary", I told her sarcastically. In 2012, Greg had finally turned his life around and found his higher power. Greg was living in Mariposa, California, helping his father, who happened to be the longest living heart transplant patient in the world. Greg's car swerved off a winding road and died instantly in the resulting crash. Greg's death made us realize how important it is to make the most of each day we have together, because life can end at any time.

We routinely watched Lifetime Movies. We always felt it was tragic when a child died, before their parents. No parent should ever have to bury their own child. Tears flowed from Joyce's eyes every time we watched a movie depicting the death of a child. Joyce and her sister have both experienced the loss of a child and it has devastated them both.

I am a Gulf War veteran who, looked at death differently, but I still reflect back on the events leading up to my mother's death during my junior year at the Naval Academy in 1975. "My mom never got to see the fruits of her labors", as tears come to my eyes and I wipe my face. "She never saw my graduation from Annapolis or even had the chance to hold any of her grandchildren."

Chapter 8 - Making Decisions

Sometimes, the solution to a problem, or a diagnosis of existing medical conditions are not obvious. Further analysis and review of symptoms and work experience allows a professional to recommend an appropriate course of action. No one asks the doctor about their grade point average. Does it matter? Are second opinions necessary?

Joyce and I had been accustomed to asking for a minimum of three bids before making a decision on home improvements. I wondered why people don't do the same when it comes to medical treatments? The cost? I laughed to myself as I reviewed my April, 2018 paycheck stub. I glanced down the list of monthly deductions, which included life insurance, disability insurance, dread disease, and a cancer policy. "Damn I spend a lot of money on insurance", I utter in a sharp tone.

"Well, it's a good thing I quit that bartender job and became a teacher with benefits." I routinely stated throughout the year. I continued to keep my promise to Peggy about Christmas. In 16 years, I never checked the credit cards or bank balances, regarding Joyce's Christmas expenditures. There was a good thing about that promise, which directly benefited our family. The bad side of this was a growing increase of credit card debt, which was creeping up each and every month.

"How did we get into so much debt?", I asked myself, after reviewing our credit card statements. Indeed, a lot of the debt we had incurred was due to my student loans, after earning three graduate degrees. That debt was justified, as it provided a steady increase to our household income, during the past 15 years.

While reviewing our debt situation, I reflected back to when we purchased a bigger home in order to accommodate the return of our adult children. Joyce was not concerned. Whenever a money problem would occur. I would always tell her, "I guess I need to make more money then. Don't worry I will figure it out," and for 16 years I have been able to do just that, one way or another. I continued to be Joyce's prince charming, in more ways than one. My ability to be there whenever she needed me was a key ingredient, which helped us overcome many obstacles, during our 16 years together.

"Don't worry honey, we can get things backs on track. I will develop a 3-year plan to get rid of our credit card debt," I told her with confidence. I continued to tell her, "We can then use my upcoming Social Security to pay these off in no time." I just wanted to collect everything I paid into the system, before my death. I remember saying to Joyce that she had the perfect retirement plan, "Me and her Social Security checks."

Chapter 9 - Somethings' Cooking

When I am not working, my hobbies are cooking or singing karaoke. My friends on Facebook always commented and say, "JB you take the world's best food porn pictures." I would routinely post pictures of my meal preparations, including before and after pics on my Enduring Classic Recipes Facebook page. Joyce loved my cooking and I loved hearing her compliments while enjoying my homemade gourmet meals, which were made with love. I always cooked by sight and smell, before I ever tasted the entrée. Joyce's daughter (Christy) made a habit of stopping by, around 5 PM to steal a taste. Her grandson Nick commented, "Jordan can make dog poop taste like an ice cream sundae. His food will make you come back over and over again."

"How am I supposed to lose any weight when he's cooking like this?", Joyce asked, as she walked into the kitchen to snoop and take a peek, at what was cooking on the stove. Joyce loved the smell and taste of a good home cooked meal, especially when I was doing the cooking. I started conducting research in order to identify foods, which might be contributing to Joyce's problems with constipation. Joyce got up one morning, in June of 2018, she looked at the scale, in disbelief, at what she was seeing. She always said, "You have to be miserable to stay skinny." The scale read 196 pounds, which meant she had lost another seven pounds, since seeing her doctor.

"Honey we need to increase your fluid and fiber intake and start to maintain data on what you consume and log the results", I told her using a teaching tone in my voice. We needed to find another way other than diarrhea every three days. After returning from Vegas, Joyce noticed she had lost ten pounds during the past month. "Wow, I may have to go buy some new clothes for when we go to Laughlin", she told me. "Yeah, right! I thought back to the summer when Joyce threw most of her clothes out, after watching the TV show What Not to Wear. "But not another $5,000 what not to wear experience please", I shouted back, as I left the master bedroom while walking down the hallway to my office.

On June 8, Joyce had another telephone appointment with her primary care doctor, who recommended another brand of laxative. I took Joyce back to urgent care on June10, with more stomach pain and the doctor gave no solution except to take more gas-x, and for her to also increase her use of laxatives.

"I've tried all of these damn laxatives and they are not working", Joyce yelled?, "Why can't they tell me what is wrong with me? I am tired of being in pain every day."

She continued to communicate via her doctor's website. As a result of those communications, her doctor ordered a CT Scan. After discovering some abnormalities, he ordered a biopsy, on the left side of Joyce's pelvic area, in order to examine her lymph nodes. This urgent procedure was performed on June 12 of 2018. Joyce complained of the rather large needle used during the procedure.

Joyce concentrated on planning for our upcoming vacation to Laughlin. We left Sunday morning for a five-day trip. I had booked a king suite, for our stay at the Aquarius Casino. Joyce was determined to go as usual, and decided to just deal with her current health problems. We still managed to have fun on this little trip.

Our best friends Barbara and Jim just happened to be in Laughlin at the same time. They were staying in a guest suite at the Riverside Casino, right next to the Aquarius. Our relationship with Barb and Jim went back 15 years. For ten of those years I was their favorite DJ for Barb's annual Halloween Party. I really enjoyed being the DJ and master of ceremonies, for these parties. I had some good times, although Joyce never liked to dress up in a costume. We still enjoyed the great food, time with friends, and an evening with our adult children.

While we were enjoying dinner, at our favorite seafood place, I took out my phone to take one of my famous food porn pictures, and posted it to Facebook. Barb was on Facebook, noticed my posting and immediately commented on my post saying, "Hey, we're at the Riverside in Laughlin." I texted back, "Great, do you guys want to get together sometime?" I quickly suggested we get together, for dinner at our Casino. "That won't work because we get free buffets here at the Riverside.", Barb sent back while complaining about the auto-correct feature on her phone.

"Ok, then let's meet after lunch, Joyce and I will walk over. How about 2:00 PM?" I quickly responded back on my new iPhone. The distance between the Riverside and Aquarius was less than 100 yards. This was normally a 5-minute walk, but because of Joyce's condition it took us forever. At that time, I decided to cut our vacation short, once again, after visiting with our friends, as I could see that Joyce was not feeling well.

Chapter 10 - The Winning Streak Ends

Barb and Jim walked back to our hotel with us so we could spend more time together. During that time, I got lucky playing the same numbers on a Keno machine left by another customer. While I was winning and cashing in tickets, Joyce was tired and went back up to our room to rest before dinner. Once again, she was hiding her pain from me. When I returned to our room, I could see the pain in her face. She could no longer hide this pain from me.

"Why didn't you tell me? Are you still constipated?", I asked her softly with anger. I assumed that she had some relief because she had been in the bathroom for over an hour that morning.

"I didn't want to worry you. You deserved to have a good time because you work so hard to provide and maintain our lifestyle. Go back and have some fun. I'm a big girl and if I really need you, I can text you or call you on your cell. `` Joyce states with confidence.

She would once again stay in our room on the third day, because she had taken magnesium citrate resulting in diarrhea once more. The pattern was set with three days of constipation and then magnesium to flush everything out. I told her, "We're going home tomorrow!"

Joyce shared an experience with me as she thinks back about her vacation trips many years ago. She told me about how she would take Nick down to the river. "Those were the days when my cousin DJ had a boat and we would go water skiing on the Colorado River", She thought out loud, with a smile on her face. "Yeah those were the days alright, but now we go to bed by 9:00 PM. We're just two old farts now. `` I responded with a chuckle.

For our past 15 years together, Joyce has defined that a true vacation must include room service. She enjoys the rattle of the wheels on the room service cart and the hot coffee thermos placed on a white tablecloth. One would think that her constipation problem might have changed the way she would normally have breakfast while on vacation.

"Can you hand me the menu", Joyce says while taking a sip of water with her evening pills.

"Do we have time for breakfast tomorrow morning before we leave" she asks.

"" Yes, I want to leave around 10 AM, do you want the usual? I asked her while packing all 12 bags we brought this time. As usual we probably took way too much stuff.

"Ok, I will have the Denver Omelet, sourdough toast, with country gravy on the side, and coffee of course. What do you want?", Joyce asks me as he takes notes to place the order.
"I'm good, I don't like to eat a lot while driving", I whisper while zipping the bags and placing them by the door of the tower suite.

The last item to be packed is my laptop. The first 13 years of our marriage I would be on the computer half the time we were on vacation, because of attending an online school. Now, I still brought my computer to check my email, in the morning, and before going to bed. I would always do a final check of the route we would travel, on my computer.

"Honey, I know we took the back route through Amboy, but I'm concerned about the lack of cell service, so unfortunately that means taking the 15 South back home", I told her. "Plus we will be closer to restroom facilities." "Sounds good to me", Joyce whispers softly, while falling asleep grasping the soft hotel pillows while grimacing in pain.

Chapter 11 – More than We Could Handle

"Did you have fun on our trip, even though we are going home early today, honey?", Joyce asked me softly, as she came out of the bathroom, after putting the final touches on her makeup.

"Yes, honey boo I did have some fun!", I told her hesitatingly, speaking half the truth. I was happy to win some money. I was unhappy because we had to cut our vacations short. Until Joyce's health improves, there would no other vacations.

"Ok, so here's the plan for today. Give me the tickets to cash in downstairs. I will call room service to bring up our breakfast. After we eat, I will call the Bellman to pick-up our luggage and then we will check out.", I said in my drill instructor tone.

Joyce says, "Aye Aye sir, and two bags full", while laughing at the same time.

"Another positive return thanks to Keno", I reminded her.

I was quiet on the way back home. Joyce kept asking me if everything was ok. "Sure", I responded and asked her if she was ok, and if we needed to stop along the way.

"I'm ok. I'll tell you if we need to stop. I love you so much," Joyce uttered. "How much?", I asked her. Joyce smiled back and says, "Bigger than the sky!" She grimaced in pain. "I just want to get home, and hopefully next week, the doctor can tell me what's going on with my body. I just want things to go back to normal." Joyce said softly, while drifting off to sleep in the front seat of our car.

"This is not just constipation. Something else is wrong!", I thought to myself as I exited Interstate 15, merging onto the 215 South, to get back home as soon as possible. I continued driving while briefly looking at the facial expressions indicating discomfort, on my wife's face as she tried to sleep.

I nudged Joyce to wake her, and asked her, "Can you call your sister, so she knows what's going on and about our coming home early. Also, ask her to move her car out of my damn garage to make it easier for me to unload the car." Joyce's sister normally parks her car in the garage when we travel on vacation.

Joyce's sister was called the bag lady by Peggy (their mother) and at the time I never understood why. During the past three years Linda stayed at our home over 360 days. Her car was fully packed with grocery bags of personal belongings, which she would bring, from Northern California. This included all of her kitchen utensils, pots and pans. She even brought her own towels, personal brand of toilet paper, and linens for the bedroom. She was also called "bossy bitch #1," because she always told people what to do even in their home. I hated the fact that she stayed in our house. I had to make changes to our lifestyle for the invading visitor. I had to make exceptions for her while she stayed with us. I was really tired of her visits, but compromised, only because of my love for Joyce. But how much was I expected to put up with?

"Damn I can't even wipe my ass with the wrong toilet paper, as long as your sister is here. This is not good for my prostate." I said with a fake smile. When people marry, the baggage that comes with the relationship may not be helpful. My personal wisdom says, "Do not burn the visiting witch at the stake until you are certain she will not be needed again."

I looked forward to being at home and back into my own kitchen. I was already planning what I wanted would cook on Sunday. I loved to grill and cook all day long. Cooking was my way of relaxing and dealing with stress. It took my mind off of many things. Sunday was not my day of rest, as several family members would seem to arrive just before dinner time. "Surprise, surprise!"

The good thing about the weekend was we didn't receive calls from doctors. I hated to pick up the phone during the week, just to hear about doctor appointments. I especially thought it was stupid to receive a voice mail message telling us to call them to make an appointment, when the office was already closed. This week even our dentist began to use a text message service and sent a text when the office was not open. During the previous 15 years, Joyce and I would only use medical insurance website, maybe once or twice a month. Little did I know that I would be using their website on a daily basis, in the not too distant future.

Chapter 12 - The Right Type of Testing

Later, during the week, after the results came back from the lab, the oncology surgeon called Joyce to inform her that he had found some abnormal tissues. He said the findings were not sufficient enough to be conclusive for a diagnosis. He stopped short of saying exactly what type of diagnosis he found inconclusive. The doctor also told Joyce that he wanted her to have another biopsy, but this time on her right side. In the meantime, we were also referred to another specialist, at the Moreno Valley Medical Center.

We should have known something was very wrong, because of the referral to the oncology/hematology department. Neither of us made a connection that it might be cancer. I was looking at this doctor as just another specialist, because of Joyce's previous skin cancer, and that somehow there might be a connection. "We need to go see an expert", I thought to myself. I could no longer tolerate her being in so much pain. My usual calm demeanor was quickly becoming impatient and the Marine inside me was about to emerge.

In the meantime, Joyce had an appointment with the oncologist on June 28, 2018. We met with the oncologist who seemed smart, intelligent, and very knowledgeable and our first impressions made us feel hopeful. On that first visit the oncologist minimized the degree of a possible cancer diagnosis, because the first biopsy had provided an insufficient prognosis of a specific type of cancer.

Later that evening I would read Joyce's entire medical record, and I discovered that the doctors feared lymphadenopathy, "CT looks like possible lymphoma." But the doctors did not share this information with us because of medical protocols. Today medical records are online, but most people do not read them. The doctor's visit summary does not tell you what the doctors are thinking as a possible diagnosis. Doctors are careful to not disclose this information without supporting evidence.

During our discussion with the oncologist I found out that this doctor was the one who actually placed an order for a second biopsy, but this time on joyce's opposite side. The second biopsy was completed on July 5, 2018. We had been trying to find out what was wrong with Joyce, for the last 90 days. We went to urgent care on July 5, and again to the emergency room on July 8, both times,because of her severe stomach and back pain.

The oncologist gave us hope in June because she told us it did not appear to be too serious and that the doctor could help get everything back under control. We would begin travelling to the Riverside and Moreno Valley Hospitals. I tried to keep all my thoughts on my job, in order to take my mind off of Joyce's health. During the next few days Joyce continued to battle with constipation, her lower back pain, along diarrhea after taking Milk of Magnesia.

On Wednesday morning, I got up at about 4:30 in the morning, a little earlier than normal. I did not sleep well because of my worries about Joyce. I got dressed as usual, grabbed the flashlight, since it was still dark and whispered, "Tommie!" I could hear the sound of Tommie's feet, while he was running through the house to the front door.   I also got up early because I was going to the school district to work on designing the next online curriculum, for the upcoming school year, in 2018-2019.

Most teachers get to enjoy their summer vacation, without thinking about work, but since earning my doctorate, I had always worked during the summer months. I was either teaching or working on designing new curriculum. I was working with Karin my coworking math teacher.

I sent a text message to Karin asking her to meet me in my classroom at 8:00 AM that morning.

Karin sent a text back, "Up again early I see. You do realize it's 5:45 AM on a vacation day, don't you? I'll meet you at 8:30 after I run an errand. How about 8:30 AM?" I texted back to her, "Okay!"

I glanced at the display on the cable box and noticed that it was now 7:40 AM. I got up and went to the kitchen and joined Joyce, who was sitting in the kitchen drinking her coffee.

I leaned over and gave Joyce a kiss, and softly said, "Honey I'm leaving in a few minutes to go work to meet Karin, can I do anything for you before I go?"

"How about a new butt hole", Joyce says while laughing.

"Ok, I'll google that to find a few for you to choose from.", I told her while chuckling back at her.

"Smart Ass!" she responds with a slight grin. "Yeah, you're right, and I have 4 college degrees to prove it. Spencer from Criminal Minds has nothing on me, except his paycheck, from his TV show. But my degrees are real. Well, I got to go", I told her as I leaned over to kiss her and tell her "I love you." Joyce utters, "Love you more!" Our dog Tommie rubs up against Joyce's leg and barks as I leave the house. Tommie always sat facing the laundry room waiting to hear the sound of the garage door going up and back down again.

Chapter 13 - The Day I Will Never Forget

July 10, 2018,is a day we shall never forget. Around 9:00 AM that morning, Joyce received a voice message from her health care provider, regarding a phone appointment with her doctor, later that afternoon. The phone rang and Joyce answered all the normal medical verification and privacy questions. Her doctor began to share information about the results of her tests, which brought tears to her eyes.

Later that day, I called home to check in with Joyce and asked her about the phone call with her doctor. she told me, "I'll tell you when you get back home." When I returned home, I knew something was very wrong. Joyce was in tears as I came through the door. Tommie was excitedly jumping on me as he always did each time I came home from work.

"What's wrong now? What did the kids do now?" I asked rather harshly. I was wondering how much one of the kids had screwed up and how much it was going to cost us this time.

"It's about me and what the doctor told me about the test results," she said while wiping tears with from her face. Joyce continued to stutter and kept weeping and could not speak. She moved from the bedroom to the kitchen table and poured herself a cup of coffee. I followed her to the kitchen and sat across the table from her. I then took her hand rubbing it slowly.

"What is it? I can take it, and I'll make the money, if needed, by working extra hours. Just tell me what it is so you can stop your crying." I told her softly.

Joyce continued to cry and began speaking between tears, "It's not fair! I finally meet the love of my life and now God is taking me away from him!" "What are you talking about? What did the doctor say?", I asked.

"He said I have lung cancer and I will need to have surgery.", Joyce uttered while still crying. "What, no Fuckin way, I yelled."

"No, this cannot be happening!', I thought to myself. We sat on the couch together, holding each other, as Joyce cried on my shoulder. I hate seeing her cry. The last time she cried so long and so hard was in May of 2013 when she got the news that her son Greg had died in a car accident.

"It's not fair, I want more time with you", she cried while holding me tightly.

"What are we going to tell the kids", she whispered to me softly. She dried her eyes and wiped her nose. My memory flashed back in time to when I received the news that my mother passed away, after only five days in the hospital, due to an aneurysm. I also remembered how nasty my relatives became by blaming my father for my mom's death. I hated that scene and the family disasters that usually come along when someone dies. Joyce was like the grandma in the movie "Soul Food." She was loved by everyone.

 "Honey we have to take this one step at a time,", I told her. What are the next steps the doctor wants us to take?"

Joyce responded, "I will have surgery, on July 17, to put a port in my chest and we have a doctor's appointment scheduled with the oncologist, in Moreno Valley on July 20. In the meantime, they have ordered a CT/PET scan, to be done in the morning of Thursday, July 20.

I reminded her, "Honey, we have a good team of doctors. They found the cancer. Let's trust them and do what they say. We can beat this cancer one more time just like before." I reassured her, while holding back my own tears.

The next few days were filled with intermittent showers of tears. We made a decision of how and when to tell the children, although we differed on our approach in telling them. We went to bed and she drifted off to sleep that night whispering, "I'm going to die." Neither one of us slept well that night. Joyce was still sitting up in bed all night, because of her lower back and stomach pains. At that time, we had no idea that constipation was a sign of lung cancer.

Over the next few days Joyce would go through many emotional ups and downs. It was unfortunate that she found out about the cancer, while she was all alone at home. There was no reason to expect this type of bad news. After all, she had just been through an annual cancer screening this past February of 2018, and she had received a clean bill of health. Both doctors saw no signs of external cancer. Why didn't they look internally for the source? For six years all of her examinations focused on the outside of her body. It was only after an internal exploratory examination that abnormalities were discovered. I started to document events and paid closer attention to my own health, because of what was now happening to Joyce.

Chapter 14 - Living During Difficult Times

During our 16 years together, Joyce and I had faced many difficult times together, but none more devastating than the events in 2013. Joyce was still working then and had to take nearly two months off for her recover, after her first cancer surgery. Her disability policy, from work, was not sufficient to replace her income.

When Joyce found out about her upcoming surgery, she started preparing a budget. Joyce was very organized and handled all of our finances. I had no interest in balancing checkbooks or dealing with finances. The last thing a math teacher wanted to do, when coming home from work, to relax, was to deal with more numbers. Although Joyce paid the bills, we made joint decisions about our expenses.

I had always been a long-term, big picture mathematician, who always tried to be pro-active in planning for our future financial needs, in case Murphy's Law would intervene and "rear its ugly head." Each year we would review and make changes to my benefits package, and the amount of deductions, to be taken out of my paycheck. I always had extra savings deducted from my check to invest in a 403 (B). Also, I would make changes to my insurance plan, based on my income.

In case I died before Joyce I wanted to make sure she would be secure for the rest of her life. In 2009, while going over our budget, Joyce was reviewing the deductions taken from my paycheck. "Jordan", she shouted while I was in the kitchen doing my husbandly duties. "Wait a minute I'm coming, I can't hear you from in here," I responded.

"What is this new charge for $109 to American Fidelity? Is this more insurance?", Joyce asked me frustratingly.

"What charge?   Oh, that's a new cancer policy that was recommended by a friend. I know we don't have cancer now, but it also pays us for routine tests we are already taking. We're not getting any younger you know", I told her.

Four years after I took out this policy, Joyce had to have cancer surgery. When she was told about her upcoming surgery, she asked me to check out that old cancer policy to see what it would pay. I went to our Living Trust file and pulled, out the insurance policy. We reviewed it together.

"Joyce, I will need you to contact the company and find out how to file a claim. It covers surgical benefits, but I don't understand this language about surgical units and an itemized bill", I told her while paging through the insurance policy. "I'll call the company tomorrow morning, because it's after 5 PM back east and they are closed," I told her.

In 2013, my communications, with insurance companies were made by telephone, mail or fax. Benefit payments would only be paid out after all the proper forms and documentation were submitted. The battle was how to get the right documentation. After I contacted the insurance company, I found out that I needed to get an itemized bill, which included the number of surgical units and then fax or express mail these documents to the insurance company's claims department.

The medical records department, for our insurance provider ,was located in Riverside, just down the street from our hospital. After Joyce's surgery, I submitted a request for her medical records. These records could be either mailed or sent to Joyce by email, as she was the patient. This process and pure hassle of getting medical records, to enable us to file a medical claim, prompted me to investigate other possibilities of streamlining this documentation process.

One of these possibilities would be to obtain a medical Power of Attorney and place it on file with our medical provider. We completed this task by creating a Living Trust. After filing her disability and insurance company paperwork we received more than enough money to cover any budget shortfalls. We are both thankful for making this smart decision regarding our cancer policy.

Joyce would never again question me regarding insurance or automatic savings deductions. My decision provided the funds which enabled us to buy our final dream home. We were just a perfect match in so many ways. I would often tell her, "What the hell was I thinking before by getting involved with or marrying any woman who did not like numbers or finance."

I thought to myself that a woman like Joyce was worth her weight in gold. It took me a long time to find her. Unfortunately, our remaining time together was uncertain. How could I ever find another lifetime match? I often thought I was too old to start over again without Joyce. I decided to focus on alternative options to help Joyce beat her cancer, once again. I was not ready to let her go!

We had a lot of time to reminiscence while waiting for her imaging test results. We discussed several questions to ask the oncologist. Our discussions about what to expect were not very serious, because of the uncertainty of the type of the possible cancer. We were hopeful it could be removed successfully, as before.

I took Joyce to her CT Scan in Riverside on July 16. Then on the morning of July 20 she had a PET scan. I decided to take her to the Red Lobster for lunch, before driving to her oncologist appointment, at the Moreno Valley medical center. The oncology department was located on the third floor in room 326, which was located all the way at the end of the hall. I drove because Joyce's vision had changed, and she had started having double vision, making it unsafe for her to drive.

We took the back roads to the hospital. The scenic route was calming and had very little traffic which took us only 45 minutes. This was a much shorter route than going to the hospital in Riverside. As we approached the hospital, I slowed down to enter the circle driveway, leading to Building 2, and found a parking space close to the building, so that Joyce would not have to walk very far. After parking I took Joyce's hand, as we entered the building for her appointment.

While in the waiting room I started to take notice of the various patients who were waiting to see the doctor. Some wore white wristbands bands, and some had on rubber stretch bandages on their arms. Some people came by themselves, while others had someone with them.

Joyce's appointment was at 2:00 PM. My stress level grew slightly, because I never liked waiting. At about 2:45 PM the nurse came out calling Joyce's name, indicating that it was her turn. She introduced herself and asked Joyce to stand on the electronic scale in order to record her weight. Then she asked Joyce what was her height? "I'm five feet 4 inches tall", Joyce said softly. The nurse took her temperature and told her 98.7. She asked Joyce to sit down, so she could take her blood pressure.

The nurse said, "Your BP is 124 over 62, that's perfect." The nurse walked us to Room#3. I held Joyce's hand to comfort her while she sat down on the examination table. It was then 3:20 pm and the doctor had still not arrived. That did not help our anxiety and frustration.

I became more and more impatient, when the doctor finally entered the room. She logged into her computer clicked a few buttons, sighed, and slowly turned to us and said, "There's no other way to say this, I'm so sorry my dear, but you have stage four lung cancer!"

Chapter 15 – Facing Death Together

After hearing the words "Stage 4 cancer", Joyce began crying and said, "I don't want to die." I composed myself after hearing that horrible diagnosis. I thought to myself, "How the hell did we go from "oh, don't worry," to stage 4 cancer in just two weeks?" "I'm so sorry dear but that is where we are," the doctor said. "I wish I had better news, but now we have some decisions to make." Joyce was still crying and asked, "How long do I have to live?"

The doctor responded, "The cancer has spread through your lymph nodes and there is a tumor in your lung, which is inoperable. Radiation is not an option at this time. We have a couple of choices, but surgery is not an option. You will have six to 18 months to live with chemo and less than six months without it. What do you want to do?"

Joyce told her, "I guess I don't have a choice. I want to spend as much time with this man that I possibly can. She turns and looks at me. It took me a long time to find him." She continued weeping and asked me. "What do you think honey? What should we do?"

I asked the doctor, "Doc, what are the different types of chemo and exactly how will this process work?" My thoughts were spinning because in ten days I had to return to work. I was wondering how we were going to handle this. I thought back about all the time we had spent, during the last three weeks going back and forth to the doctor appointments. Now we understood the reason for her emergency surgery was to place an intravenous port into her chest. The port was now showing as a big half-dollar lump on the left side of Joyce's chest.

The doctor discussed the differences between chemo and immunotherapy. She explained in detail why radiation and surgery were not options, because the disease was already metastatic and was quickly spreading to unspecified areas of her body. After a joint discussion, we made the decision to begin chemo treatments, based on the doctor's recommendation.

The hematology nurse explained about the pre-chemo class which would explain the do's and don'ts during chemo treatments. She also described the cycle of once every three weeks, with a combo of two different chemo prescriptions and a saline flush before and after each infusion. Because of my work schedule we requested that the infusions be on Monday afternoons. The doctor told us we would receive a call for appointment dates and times. The plan was to do 9 weeks, or three cycles of chemo followed by a CT scan to see if it was working. Each chemo infusion would take place every three weeks. The nurse gave me some reading materials to take home.

Our life together would never be the same after this moment. We would have many more difficult times to come. During all our previous doctor appointments we had routinely thrown away the medical report called a visit summary. Now, I began to read each summary thoroughly. It was like reading a foreign language. No more could I simply leave everything up to medical personnel, as the only experts regarding Joyce's health and welfare.

I would tear up whenever I thought about watching Joyce prepare her pill box every week, during the past six years. At the time I had no idea what medications she was taking or why. I knew she was a Type 2 diabetic, taking pills and insulin shots. I vividly remembered all the pills she had been taking each day. I hadn't given it a second thought, because Joyce seemed to be doing fine.

When we got back home, I went to the master bathroom and picked up each bottle to read them. Joyce was still capable of fixing her own pill box and that would remain, for now. I knew that at some point I would have to take over that responsibility as well. I would need help trying to balance work and taking care of Joyce. Unfortunately, that would end our privacy as Joyce would now require someone to help her during the day.

I was not looking forward to sharing the details of my summer vacation, when returning to school, because now Joyce and I would be facing death together.

Chapter 16 – Living Trustfully

In 2005, Joyce helped her Mom create a Living Trust, so that they could prepare in advance for what could happen with her estate. Joyce created the document herself and then had it notarized. She then became the executor of Peggy's estate, upon her death. We created our own Living Trust in 2012, and then modified and updated it after moving into our 55+ retirement community, in 2017. Our trust contained both of our Wills, our Power of Attorneys, and the final distribution of assets, in the event of both of our deaths.

After receiving the devastating new, in 2018, regarding Joyce's cancer diagnosis, we spent the next few days reviewing and making changes to our Trust. Joyce pulled out her budget sheet and prepared a budget based on our current expenses, excluding her income. The next thing we did was to call a representative from Miller Jones Mortuary to discuss and make final arrangements, for both of us.. This process helped to ease our minds. This preplanning would help make a smooth transition and eliminate any financial hardship on the surviving spouse.

When Joyce's mom died, about eleven years ago, Joyce gained invaluable experience and insight into how to deal with the Social Security Administration and insurance companies. She knew that benefit payments would take a while and so it was best to plan ahead. As a result of this experience we set-up different policies for different reasons. We had four different purposes for our life insurance policies:

1. Six months of expense income (Whole Life Level Payment)

2. Funeral Expenses (Term - AARP)

3. Liquidation of Credit Card Debt and Emergency Fund (Life Insurance Term)

4. Mortgage Deduction (Life Insurance Term)

In addition to our insurance policies, I was adamant about maintaining up to six months of expenses in our savings and investment accounts, which would be readily accessible. All these precautions were put in place, because of our previous personal experiences, involving the death of our parents, and their final affairs. Now, it was time for us to make decisions and do the same for ourselves. At least we had time to talk things over, instead of having to deal with a sudden death. The doctor gave Joyce 6-18 months to live, with chemotherapy. There were no guarantees, as her cancer had already spread to multiple locations in her body.

 "So how do we tell the family", Joyce asked. I responded, "Let's have a BBQ and invite the kids, who live close enough to come. We can call the rest of them, but not all at once. We still have time." After a brief discussion that's what we chose to do. So, we gathered our family together and after we ate an enjoyable meal, we sat everyone down in the living room to share the bad news. They were all in shock, as we were when the doctor broke the news to us. We then called the rest of the family during the next few days.

I called my co-worker Karin and asked her to inform the school principal and district administration. I did not want to keep repeating our story over and over again. I would eventually have to share the news with my students, with whom I had developed a strong bond, over the last two years. They needed to be aware that their professor would be absent more than usual, during the next years to come.

During the discussions with our family, Joyce explained the course of action to be taken regarding her treatments. She would be taking these treatments for the next few months. We also identified the help that would be necessary during this difficult time.

Because I was a literal working demon, I had accumulated a lot of sick leave hours and personal necessity leave. However, I was mindful not to abuse my work perks. I sat down with my school principal and promised to keep him informed of any changes that might impact my ability to perform my responsibilities. He was very supportive, as he previously had a similar experience in battling cancer with his son.

On Monday morning, after telling our family we drove to attend a chemo education class. During this education class we learned about the many side effects with chemo and the additional medications that needed to be taken before and after each treatment. The initial dose of chemo would be administered once every three weeks. A CT scan needed to be taken at the beginning and after each 9-week cycle. Blood work needed to be taken 1-2 days before each treatment, as well. A visit to the doctor would happen at the beginning and end of each cycle. There would be a total of ten visits to the hospital for each cycle.

"If her appointments for treatment were scheduled after 2:00 PM, they wouldn't interfere with my work schedule," I told her while pushing her wheelchair down the hall, on our way to the parking lot.

"We can get help from Christy and Lynn said she would drive back down from Northern California to help", Joyce said while getting into the car.

"At least I have you. Do you know how much I love you?" Joyce told me as she squeezed my hand as tears ran down her face on our drive back home.

We would find out later that we were not alone in our battle with cancer. Many of our friends and associates were currently, or in the past, in a similar situation with members of their families. This network of friends and co-workers, as fellow survivors of cancer, would prove to be very helpful and provide solutions to many of our challenges during the next several months. If not for our marriage she would have been all alone to deal with this terminal illness. She was not alone anymore. She had the full support of a loving husband. Most importantly she would not die alone.

Chapter 17 - The Battle Against Cancer Begins

Joyce's first aggressive chemo treatment began 21 days after her initial diagnosis. Time goes by quickly, but not as quickly as you would like it to go, when your loved one was dying from cancer. The oncology department was always packed, on a daily basis. We soon discovered many people were going through the same situation. We learned to expect delays in getting orders for additional tests, imagery, and radiation treatments. We also, learned to be especially careful when obtaining outside referrals to other medical facilities, or doctors outside our provider network.

The sharing of information from one medical provider to the another was not a smooth transaction and could cause unnecessary delays in receiving treatments. The average time to get an appointment for a CT scan was 10 days. The process of switching between chemo and radiation treatments was six weeks. We were advised to have someone take Joyce to her first treatments, as it was not known what side effects she might experience.

Upon hearing the news about Joyce's diagnosis, her sister Lynn volunteered to return to Hemet and help with her care. When Joyce's phone rang she quietly said "Hello", while motioning and whispering to me it's my sister. When she got off the phone, she told me that her sister was on her way and would arrive three days before her next chemo education class.   Linda would now take over driving Joyce to her chemo education classes, which allowed me to attend an important preschool workshop.

Lynn has had a lifetime habit of taking forever to get ready to go anyplace. Joyce often joked that her daughter Christy must have been Linda's child, as they both took about three hours to get ready to go anywhere. I would often tell them that we had to be somewhere at least an hour before we had to be there, so they would not be late.   The night before her appointment, Joyce reminded her sister that they needed to leave by 11:00 AM tomorrow morning.

Lynn is an organic food freak and an herbal holistic enthusiast. She eats the same healthy breakfast and then takes her dog Whitney, for a walk before going anywhere. At 8:30 after finishing her breakfast Linda said to Whitney, "Are you ready to go to the park? We'll be going in just a few minutes. Mommy loves you so much." "I'm taking Whitney to the park" she yelled to Joyce. "What time is your appointment again?", she asked. Joyce thought to herself, "How many times do I need to tell the bitch, #%##@@@@." Once again Joyce told her "12:30." "I'll be right back," Linda told her while going out the front door. Joyce looked at the clock noting the time was now 9:15 AM. That morning Joyce was ready and sat impatiently in her room, ready to go by 10:00 AM. She thought to herself, "we need to leave by 11:00 AM because I need to be there 15 minutes before my appointment. I should have lied about the correct appointment time."

Lynn finally returned and now the time is 10:10 AM. "I'm going to take my shower and get ready," Linda told Joyce. Joyce thought to herself, "that's going to take over an hour." Lynn came out of the bathroom, with her hair in a towel, and steam flowing out of the guest bathroom so much that it sets off the smoke alarm. She was frantic as she opened the front door and got another towel and flapped it through the air. Meanwhile the dogs were yapping, running around in circles.

Joyce asked her, "Who's driving?" Linda quickly responded, "I'll drive." After all the excitement was over, it was then 11:15 AM and Joyce was waiting in the kitchen. She yelled to Lynn, "We have to go. We're going to be late!" "Ok, ok…." Lynn replied. They finally left at 11:25 AM.

Lynn never drove the speed limit and she never used navigation. Somehow, miraculously they arrive at 12:35 PM, a new world's record.

Although, Linda is a health nut, some of her advice (always an order never a suggestion) was practical and helpful. I was on edge because she already spends 3 months out of every year living at our house. And now, we must once again change our living routine to accommodate her. This situation would not last much longer, as I had already had enough. Once again, I had to concede because I also needed her to help care for Joyce. When Linda was in town, I made a habit of pouring myself into my work, so I didn't have to spend much time with her.

After returning home from work that day, I asked them about the doctor's appointment. Linda is in the kitchen preparing something for Whitney to eat. There were bags of groceries on the kitchen counters and the kitchen trashcan was full of discarded food that Linda had removed from our refrigerator, once again never bothering to ask permission. Of course, the trash was stacked by the door waiting for me to take it outside.

Linda handed me a stack of papers and said you need to read these. As I read the first few pages, I thought to myself, "The list for what we couldn't do was much longer than what we could do." Now I understood why Linda threw-out so many items from the refrigerator. Joyce's diet was going to change dramatically. I was going to have to learn how to cook for cancer. Yuck! She's going to hate that!

I took Joyce to the first her chemo treatment the next day. Her cycle for chemo treatment included two different chemicals which were infused through the port in her chest. At the end of each cycle her doctor ordered a CT Scan to check the progress of the original cancer. If the treatment impeded the cancer growth, then the meds would stay the same. Joyce went two nine-week cycles, with the same chemo until it stopped working. Her doctor would then change to a different type of chemo infusion. There were side effects and the big one for Joyce was she could no longer be able to taste my good cooking.

Chapter 18 - Side Effects

Chemotherapy is one form of treatment for lung cancer. This drug has many side effects. These side effects, vary from one type of drug to another and depending on the number of treatments given.

Treatments have changed over the past few years. There is not just one medication for chemo. Chemo is very expensive, as our itemized bill from the health care provider indicated. Each treatment had a cost of $20,000. Fortunately, Joyce's side effects were minimal. In the beginning she was given preventive medications for nausea and vomiting, which worked perfectly throughout her treatments.

Joyce's chemo treatments became a routine that merged into our already busy lifestyle. She knew that I loved her, but that also bothered her from time to time. She told me over and over again if she could just get rid of the back pain and constipation, she could deal with everything, else even losing her hair. But the pain in her stomach and lower back was impacting our intimacy together. Some of the other patients, we had encountered in the waiting rooms, shared that individual side effects could usually be dealt with, but it was difficult when so many side effects occurred at the same time. Some people have chemotherapy on an out-patient basis, while others need to stay in the hospital. Thank goodness Joyce's treatments were on an outpatient basis.

Her chemo drugs were given through the port in her chest. These treatments consisted of 2 bags of chemo and one bag of saline. The first step was to connect the port using saline to backwash to see if blood was present in the syringe, before administering the chemo. After several treatments Joyce's nurses were unable to produce a blood backwash, and therefore the rest of her chemo treatments had to be done intravenously. She had lost nearly 40 pounds over the last year and her veins were now more accessible. Chemo treatments were not a problem for Joyce, as she was able to relax in a nice lounge chair and read one of her favorite books. She was an avid reader and reading helped her to relax, during her 3-hour treatments.

Joyce told her nurses, she was now experiencing pain, which felt like pins and needles being stuck in her fingers and hands. She experienced very little hair loss and began to go back to her hairdresser, and to get her nails done.

Joyce told me that chemotherapy made her feel physically tired and sometimes depressed. From time to time, she also commented on a temporary loss of smell and taste.

I could always tell when she was feeling really good, because she would go shopping and spend more time with the kids. When she began shopping for Christmas, I knew she must have really felt good! After her first cycle of chemo she began shopping and packages began to pile up in the closets, once again. "She's back!", I thought to myself.

Chapter 19 - It's Not Over

J oyce continued her chemo treatments for three more cycles. She was administered Carboplatin and Pemetrexed. The amount of her pain continued to persist. She was holding up well, but I continued to have concerns, because nothing had stopped the persistent constipation problems, which affected our quality of life. Joyce continued to sit up in bed during the night. She was managing herself well during the day. The doctor requested an MRI to determine if there were any issues with her brain, which might be causing her double vision. But Joyce freaked out when she went to take the MRI exam. I was angry with the technician, because I was not allowed to be with and comfort her during the imagery test. I would not let that happen again.

Joyce was unable to drive for next the three months. A visit to the optometrist found a solution by prescribing a new set of coke bottle lenses for her glasses. I remembered laughing about a girl who wore similar glasses like these, when I was in grade school. I now understood why that little girl had those glasses and that made me very sad. Her glasses were necessary to improve her quality of life.

After four chemo cycles, her CT Scan did not show a decrease in the size of her tumors. The doctor removed the Carboplatin treatment, for the next few cycles. In the meantime, Joyce developed a swelling in her left leg, with severe Edema and Cellulitis. Meanwhile her constipation and stomach pain had not improved. After three months she was referred to a gastrointestinal specialist. Her sister Lynn was now back in town and took Joyce to her next appointment on, Dec 13, 2018. This office visit lasted about five minutes and ended with Joyce's doctor giving her a prescription for Amitiza. This drug was not covered by our insurance provider. Joyce was shocked when she was told out the out of pocket cost would be $400. She walked out of the hospital refusing to buy the medication.

When I called her to find out what happened, I was upset and told her to go back and get the medicine. I didn't care what it cost. I just wanted her to feel normal, once again. This medication gave her some relief from the constipation, but unfortunately gave her extreme stomach pain.

Later that evening, on Dec 18, the oncologist conducted a telephone visit with Joyce, and told her the chemo was not working, and would require a new course of action. Joyce decided she wanted to try immunotherapy. The oncologist then gave her a referral for radiation treatment, because there was evidence of a lymph node blockage, which was causing the swelling in her legs. The next day (Dec 19) we drove to Ontario and met with the radiation doctor. We discussed the treatment location options and decided to use an outside referral to the City of Hope, in Wildomar (25 miles away). This shorter commute would be more comfortable for both of us.

Joyce was struggling with her pain, but we were able to hold our annual Christmas Eve party. She was so happy that night even though she was in a lot of pain. We were not able to have a Christmas dinner that year because she needed to rest. Her daughter and grandkids stayed the night, so they could be with Joyce in the morning and open presents with us.

It took two weeks before Joyce could be seen by the City of Hope doctor (Dec 31). And after the initial office visit, the nurse told me they had not received the digital imagery from my medical provider. This was a big problem! Their doctor confirmed that radiation should help reduce the swelling in Joyce's legs. I spent the next few days tracking down the medical release of information and finally out of frustration, I drove 120 miles to deliver a copy of Joyce's CD containing her imaging files. I registered a complaint to our health care provider about the poor service. A customer service representative contacted me and apologized for the inconvenience. After the City of Hope consultation Joyce had to undergo another digital scan to specifically mark the areas for her radiation treatments. She was scheduled for 15 treatments, which would run on consecutive days, except for the weekends. Radiation and immunotherapy were now being done simultaneously. The immunotherapy would now be done on Monday afternoon and the radiation treatments ,for Monday mornings. She would go to lunch between treatments and spend quality time with her family. By the end of February Joyce's legs and feet had returned to normal and she could actually get back to wearing her shoes, and walking normally.

Doctors don't always see obvious signs of cancer with an external examination. Cancer does not just grow externally. A complete internal examination should be done. Doctors should also explore and search for additional symptoms or signs of cancer. A Carcinoembryonic Antigen Test (CEA) should also be conducted. This test measures a protein called CEA in the blood. People with cancer have higher than normal levels of this protein. The CEA test results can help your doctor discover if the cancer is growing, and whether your treatment is working. Secretly, Joyce's doctor had been looking at this test to determine if the chemo was working. The normal level for this test is less than 5 nanograms per milliliter (<=5.0 ng/ml). As of April 5, 2019, Joyce's value was 554 ng/ml. By May it had increased to over 600 ng/ml, indicating, that the cancer was spreading rapidly. May 20, 2019 was her last immunotherapy treatment. Her doctor ordered another MRI on May 22.

This time I took time off from work, to provide her comfort and support. The doctor ordered a prescription of Ativan to be taken right before her test, to reduce her anxiety and fear.

On May 23, we met with her oncologist, who informed us that her cancer had spread to her brain. Once more, she referred Joyce for radiation. It took 12 days to obtain an office appointment for brain radiation. During that time the cancer had spread from six to 11 spots in her brain. As a result, the radiation specialist recommended a whole brain radiation. She then gave us another referral, to the City of Hope.

We began to look for holistic treatments. Joyce' constipation was now chronic, and the $400 pills were not working, and she refused to take them anymore. After eight months of infusion she was still getting very tired. After a recommendation from my cousin, I purchased CBD products for Joyce. She began to take CBD oil drops to help with her anxiety,and began using a CBD sleep support, in order to get a good night's sleep. Her sister and daughter convinced her to start using THC vape for her pain. We were desperate for solutions to ease her pain.

At the time I disagreed with her using pot. But my hands were tied. The daily regimen of morphine was not working, and she continued to wake up in the middle of the night, in pain. Her lack of sleep was beginning to impact my ability to go to work each mornings. Although, THC is legal in California as a recreational drug, I did not like how it affected and disoriented her. At that time, I told her I would be taking over the bills, as long as she was using marijuana.

Although her daughter and sister loved Joyce, it was hard for them to understand they were not in charge. I was responsible for her health insurance and I had medical Power of Attorney. It was my decision, only, to decide what care Joyce would receive. I had to kick her sister out of our house, before this battle with cancer would end. A very loud argument with Joyce's sister would end my 1000 days of living under her organic captivity. She would never return to stay at our home again. I would now take care of Joyce by myself, and seek additional help from friends and other family members.

Chapter 20 – The Disease Spreads

The long wait continued and finally Joyce had an appointment with the City of Hope specialist. We met with him on June 24, 2019, one month after the referral from our medical provider. Our appointment was at 1:30 PM. We arrived early at 1:00 PM, but the doctor did not see us until 1:55 PM. After our office visit, I went to check out with the receptionist, and was informed, that once again, the referral authorization had been worded incorrectly. This was a "he said she said" issue and this time I was really pissed. I registered a complaint all the way up the chain, until our medical provider assigned me to an expediter.

A radiation doctor from Los Angeles convinced us to seek treatment from the radiation center in Ontario, CA. I reluctantly agreed with her, and vowed never to use an outside provider again. After a wait of six weeks Joyce's radiation treatment began on July 3rd, 2019. Her image treatment plan, and her first radiation treatment, would take place on the, same day resulting in immediate treatment.

The first stage of treatment was a planning image scan, and in this case, the making of a facial mask for her whole brain radiation. I could not be in the room to support her during the first appointment. After 20 minutes the nurse came out to get me to help calm Joyce down. As a result, they asked me to remain in the examination waiting room. She was terrified, they were placing this fencing-like mask over her entire head. She persevered and after four tries the nurse was able to complete the facial mask.

The reason I requested the outside referral was because the route from the Moreno Valley facility was dangerous and I could not imagine driving it for 11-15 days in a row. I was now 65 years old and still considered myself a very good defensive driver. Since the beginning of the year, I had taken over the driving duties. I found an alternative route to drive to the Ontario radiation center.

Our customer service improved dramatically, after my official complaints. Now, without having to ask, the receptionist automatically provided me with a medical report that my cancer insurance company would accept. Joyce became weaker after her seventh treatment. She would fall asleep often. She would sometimes go to the bathroom and fall asleep on the toilet.

Joyce became disoriented and was losing her balance, which made it difficult for her to walk by herself. I then purchased a wheelchair to take her to and from the hospital. Many times there were no wheelchairs to be found. She had a new ride and she loved it. When you have someone with mobility issues it becomes difficult to get them to the hospital unless you own your own equipment. I thought to myself, "Thank God for that Cancer Policy!"

That cancer policy paid mileage benefits for any trips exceeding 100 miles. I originally bought the policy, because of the cash reimbursement benefits. We were excited to discover the policy paid much more than preventative services. Our cancer policy provided for a quality of life, when it was most needed. Not every family is prepared to handle traumatic events, or deal with the hurt, pain and suffering of a loved one, with a terminal illness.

Chapter 21 – Nothing is What It Seems– July 2019

From April 2018, to July 2019, we would take 90+ trips to a medical facility for doctor visits, urgent care, emergency care, blood tests, and lab work. There would be an additional 57 trips for chemo and immunotherapy, and radiation treatments. A total of 147 visitations to medical facilities, in less than one year. Before the spread of cancer Joyce had only gone to the doctor about three to four times a year. I would also routinely schedule blood work and a physical for myself, during breaks from school. We would both try to make our appointments for the same day, since we shared the same primary care doctor for the past 15 years.

Besides the problems with constipation and lower back pain, Joyce also had problems with edema in both of her legs, two different times. The first time was over the Christmas holidays (2018) and the second was at the beginning of May (2019), which resulted in Joyce's legs becoming infected, with edema. The first time the doctor tried treating her with water pills (Lasix) which did not work. The second time the emergency room doctor prescribed antibiotics, due to her pending radiation treatment.

It was now June and I was finally on summer vacation. During the wait for radiation treatments I was able to spend a lot of personal time with Joyce. I was finally able to see, first-hand, the amount of pain she was suffering each day.

When Joyce heard the news about her brain cancer, she was even more focused on taking one more vacation trip together. She felt this would be our last opportunity, to do so. We had not been on a vacation for over a year. She shared her plans with me, while waiting for our next appointment, with our medical provider. Joyce told them that no further treatment would start until after we returned from vacation.

So, I finally gave in and we planned a vacation to Vegas and Laughlin. We again stayed at our favorite hotels. Joyce hid her pain well for the first part of our vacation in Vegas. As we left for Laughlin Joyce was in serious pain, but she did not share that fact with me.

She had purchased THC vape before leaving, to help hide her pain. But she was cautious about using it in a non-smoking room for fear of setting off the smoke alarm. She also had a CBD vape, which helped to relieve her pain and anxiety. By the time we reached Laughlin she had been constipated for four days. She was on morphine and taking up to six Norco a day. Nothing was working. The main reason for this was because she had stopped taking the steroids her doctor had prescribed. I was unaware of this until I checked her medical case and found the discrepancy. From that point forward, I took charge of her medications. I did not allow her to take anything from anyone without my knowledge. We had watched enough Lifetime movies to know I would be the first person under suspicion upon her death. Needless to say, I cut the vacation trip short, once again leaving our beautiful Majestic Suite overlooking the Colorado River.

When we returned home, I reviewed all her medications. I organized them and used my math knowledge to calculate when her pain would take place. I recorded data for five consecutive days, and was then able to predict when she would be in pain again, within plus or minus (+/-) 30 minutes. Using this information, I sent a message to her doctor explaining that the frequency of Joyce's dosage for morphine needed to be changed. Under her doctor's guidance, I experimented with the frequency and dosage, a little at a time, until I successfully eliminated her pain for three consecutive days. After reporting the findings to her oncologist, she changed and updated Joyce's morphine prescription. Next, I began to collect data on her bowel movement activity.

I became concerned that Joyce was in her final days, for sure. It was just a matter of time. I obtained copies of her medical records. I filed for accelerated benefits, in order to execute the terminal illness clause, of her life insurance policies. I realized that throughout this whole experience, I had never read any of the doctor notes or summaries in detail. I received an encrypted file that contained her past two years of medical records. Upon reading the first few pages I was astonished to discover a flaw in the files regarding her doctor's instructions for laxatives.

After combing through her medical reports, I discovered that Joyce was given verbal instructions, which did not match the directions in her medical files. I knew this to be true, as I was there at each visit since her cancer diagnosis. I found the directions on the laxative stated to take up to 4 tablets two times a day instead of only one tablet twice a day. I found the directions for MOM or Milk of Magnesia was to take 15ml twice a day, every day, to relieve constipation in addition to stool softeners. I then placed her back on this regimen. I made an improvement in reducing her constipation problems. Since making those changes Joyce's quality of life improved.

Analysis of Medical Records

I moved a computer to our master bedroom to help take better care of Joyce. I poured all my time into reading every detail about her health. I was embarrassed. I did not know the gravity of everything that was going on, and now I was pretty pissed off. I discovered outright lies, and misstatements by nurses and doctors, within her medical records. Some were unintentional or maybe mistakes, but some were simply made to "cover their asses". I decided to take action and continued to collect data to end Joyce's constipation problems.

After reading Joyce's medical records, I noticed her doctors had not shared all of her test results. For instance, the CEA cancer marker test results were not revealed, until my discovery, and then only after repeated requests for the information from her oncologist. The test results of her CEA blood test in May of 2019, were verbally shared, but not automatically released. In fact, during the past four years, my own PSA blood test results were only available from the doctor. The next thing I discovered about our health care provider was that I gave up my right to sue any medical professional and could only seek arbitration to settle differences or malpractice. The good news was that other than the written inaccuracies I was still pretty happy with my overall medical care. This life experience of facing death with Joyce, caused me to be more vigilant and aware, when reviewing medical summaries, before signing them. I would now annually review our benefits from each insurance policy.

Chapter 22 – The Language of Cancer

I am a teacher of mathematics and an expert in modifying instructional methods. I provide my students with an opportunity to learn, by using a rigorous curriculum and instruction, no matter the extent of their learning disability. After 15 years of instruction I figured out that the language of mathematics was one of the most critical stumbling blocks to learning. Students must be taught the language of math to make connections, by using different methods (math representations) in order to develop, solidify and practice their understanding of math concepts.

A patient who reads their doctor's notes, after each office visit, or views pathology reports are at a disadvantage and may have difficulty understanding the content, because of medical notations, abbreviations, and the overall structure of medical terms. An attempt to decipher this information should remind people of why it takes so long for a person to earn a doctorate degree. I began my experience as a doctoral researcher by conducting a review of literature to understand key medical vocabulary, which would give me a better understanding of cancer terminology.

When I began reviewing Joyce's past after-visit summaries, I noticed at the top of each report there were two tabs and one of them was for notes. After clicking this tab, I discovered a world of new information. I printed out the complete visitation summary and underlined what was important and circled all medical terms. Like most people I began my research by using Google to search for the definition of terms I did not understand. What follows in this chapter are only a few of the terms that helped me understand Joyce's cancer and what it was doing to her body. You will find a list of terms at the end of this book, which I found helpful. This chapter will also provide a few examples of medical terms that were important to me and helped deepen my understanding of Joyce's medical condition and prognosis for her recovery.

Once you have been diagnosed with cancer, your doctor will tell you what stage you are in. This diagnosis will describe the size of your cancer and how far it has spread. Cancer is typically labeled in stages from one (I) to four (IV), with four (IV) being the most serious (terminal). These broad groups are based on a much more detailed system, which includes specific information about the tumor (size, type, location) and how it affects the rest of your body. It's important to understand your cancer stage for several reasons:

Treatment: It helps your doctor decide which treatment will work best. An early-stage cancer may call for surgery, while an advanced-stage cancer may need chemotherapy, immunotherapy, or radiation.

Outlook: Your recovery will depend, in part, on how early your cancer is discovered. Your stage gives you an idea of your possible outcome.

Research: Most hospitals work with a national database ,which keeps track of the treatments used, and how well they will work. Researchers can compare similar cases to find the most effective treatments.

Most cancers that involve a tumor are staged in five broad groups. These are usually referred to with Roman numerals. Other kinds, like blood cancers, lymphoma, and brain cancer, have their own staging systems. They all will tell you how advanced your cancer is. The stages are listed below:

- **Stage zero (0)** means there's no cancer, only abnormal cells with the potential to become cancer. This is also called **carcinoma** in situ.
- **Stage One (I)** means the cancer is small and only in one area. This is also called early-stage cancer.
- **Stage Two and Three (II and III)** means the cancer is larger and has grown into nearby tissues or lymph nodes.
- **Stage Four (IV)** means the cancer has spread to other parts of your body. It's also called invasive, advanced or metastatic cancer.

Joyce was diagnosed with stage 4 lung cancer, metastatic to unspecified sites on July 10, 2018. Her type of cancer was named after where the primary source tumor was located. Metastatic means the cancer is invasive and has spread to other parts of her body. Joyce previously had anal and vulvar cancer (Stage I) in the outside tissue, which was accessible and extractable by surgery. Invasive cancer is cancer that has spread beyond the layer of tissue in which it developed and is growing into surrounding, healthy tissues. Also called infiltrating cancer.

The statement of stage 4 diagnosis is not sufficient for the patient or the family to conceptualize what that really means. The family needs to review their doctor's notes and closely read their pathology reports. A physical exam and several tests are used to determine your clinical stage -- an estimate of how far your cancer has spread. Tests may include blood and other lab tests and imaging scans. Those may be X-rays or any of the following:

Magnetic resonance imaging (MRI): Powerful magnets and radio waves are used to make detailed images of the affected area.

Computerized Tomography (CT) scan: Several X-rays are taken from different angles and put together to show more information.

Ultrasound: High-frequency sound waves are used to make images of the inside of your body.

Joyce had two biopsies, in which a small piece of tissue was taken and then examined under a microscope. If a tumor is removed by surgery, a doctor may discover and learn more about it and how it has affected your body. That information will be added to your test results to determine your pathologic stage, or surgical stage. This can be different from the cancer'sclinical stage, and it's considered more accurate. During the last year of her life Joyce had received all of the above tests, during the treatment of her terminal illness.

In retrospect it is very important to complete an MRI of the brain very early when beginning treatment for metastatic stage 4 cancer. Do not wait to get this test done!

Chapter 23 - Understanding the Signs of Cancer and Treatments

Cancer is a relentless disease that takes on many forms. The type of cancer is named after the original location in the body. Joyce's diagnosis was lung cancer, due to many years of smoking.

There are many types of cancer treatments. The types of treatment a person receives will depend on the type of cancer they have and how advanced it is. Some people with cancer will have only one treatment. But most people have a combination of treatments, such as surgery with chemotherapy and/or radiation therapy. If you need treatment for cancer, you will have a lot to learn and think about.

It is normal to feel overwhelmed and confused. But, talking with your doctor and learning about the types of treatments, which are available may help you feel more in control. There are many questions you will need to ask your doctor, at different times, during your treatment. Family members taking charge of your care need to become familiar with all of the informational pamphlets you will receive, before the first treatment. If you have a third-party cancer insurance policy, then you will need to find out how to obtain copies of itemized billing statements, once treatment begins, in order to file claims for benefits. If you are close to a facility, then you can drive and get the copies easily. In our case we would have to drive over 100 miles round trip. American Fidelity allows you to file claims online. You will need a printer with scanner functions. It will also be advantageous to have a dedicated land line connected to a fax machine.

The following were the different treatments made available to Joyce during her battle against cancer.

• Surgery was used to install a port for infusion of chemotherapy.

• Radiation therapy was used for precision treatment that uses high doses of radiation to kill cancer cells and shrink tumors.

• Chemotherapy was a type of cancer treatment that uses drugs to kill cancer cells.

• Immunotherapy was a type of treatment that helped her immune system fight cancer.

Individuals with hazard factors for malignant growth (for instance, smokers, substantial liquor use, high sun presentation, hereditary qualities) ought to be intensely mindful of potential disease manifestations and be assessed annually by their doctor. The ideal approach to battle malignant growths is by aversion (disposing of or diminishing danger factors) and early identification. The use of malignant growth treatments have progressed each year, and along with early recognition, has made numerous tumors treatable. Subsequently, you will need to know which side effects may point to cancer. Individuals ought not to disregard a recurring symptom.

What Are Signs and Symptoms of Cancer?

Cancer offers the vast majority of people no manifestations or hints. Tragically, every grumbling or side effect of cancer can also be clarified by an innocuous condition. A few diseases happen much of the time in particular age groups. On the off chance specific indications arise, a specialist should be seen, for further assessment. Please consult a qualified medical professional, if any of these symptoms occur. Some vital signs that may emerge with cancer are as follows:

Persistent hack or blood-tinged salivation

• These side effects more often than not speak to uncomplicated contaminations, for example, bronchitis or sinusitis.
• They could be side effects of lung cancer or head and neck cancer. Anybody with a bothering hack that keeps going over a month or with blood in the bodily fluid that is hacked up should see a specialist.

A change in gut propensities (bowel movements)

• Most changes in gut propensities are identified with your eating routine and liquid consumptions.

• In some cases, doctors may see pencil-dainty stools with colon cancer.

• Occasionally, cancer displays constant looseness of the bowels.

• Some individuals with infection feel as though they need defecation and still feel that need after they have had a stable discharge. On the off chance that any of these abnormal side-effects last more than a couple of days, they require assessment.

• Any critical change in entrail propensities (bowel movements) that can't be conclusively clarified by dietary changes could be cancer-related and should be assessed.

Blood in the stool

• A specialist consistently ought to research blood in your stool.

• Hemorrhoids much of the time cause rectal dying, but since hemorrhoids are so healthy, they may exist with cancer. In this way, notwithstanding when you have hemorrhoids, you ought to have a specialist look at your whole intestinal tract when you have blood in your solid discharges.

• With a few people, X-beam studies might be sufficient to explain a determination.

• Colonoscopy is typically prescribed. Routine colonoscopy, even without manifestations, is prescribed once you are 50 years of age.

Unexplained paleness (low blood tally)

• Anemia is a condition wherein individuals have less than the average number of red platelets in their blood. Iron deficiency ought to consistently be researched.

• There are numerous sorts of frailty, yet blood misfortune quite often causes iron inadequacy sickliness. Except if there is an essential wellspring of continuous blood misfortune, this paleness should be clarified.

• Many cancers can cause pallor, however inside tumors most normally cause iron inadequacy sickliness. Assessment ought to incorporate endoscopy or X-beam investigations of your upper and lower intestinal tracts.

Breast bump or bosom release

•   Most bosom lumps are non-cancerous tumors, for example, fibroadenomas or blisters. In any case, all breast irregularities should undergo screening for the likelihood of bosom cancer.

•   A negative mammogram result isn't ordinarily adequate to assess a bosom knot. Your primary care physician needs to decide the fitting X-beam study, which may incorporate an MRI or an ultrasound of the bosom.

•   Generally, finding requires a needle yearning or biopsy (a little tissue test).

•   Discharge from a bosom is healthy, yet a few types of discharge might be indications of cancer. If the spill is wicked or from just a single areola, further assessment is prescribed.

•   Women are encouraged to direct month to month bosom self-assessments.

Lumps in the testicles

•   Most men (90%) with cancer of the gonad have an effortless or awkward protuberance on a gonad.

•   Some men have an augmented gonad.

•   Other conditions, for example, contaminations and swollen veins, can likewise cause changes in your gonads, yet any protuberance ought to be assessed.

•   Men are encouraged to lead a month to month testicular self-assessments.

A Change in Urinary Habits (Pee)

• Urinary indications can incorporate successive pee, modest quantities of pee, and moderate pee stream or a general change in bladder work.

• These indications can be brought about by urinary contaminations (for the most part in ladies) or, in men, by an expanded prostate organ.

• Most men will experience the ill effects of innocuous prostate broadening as they age and will frequently have these urinary side effects.

• These indications may likewise flag prostate cancer.

• Men encountering urinary indications need further examination, potentially including blood tests and an advanced rectal test. The PSA blood test, its signs, and elucidation of results ought to be talked about with your human services supplier.

• If cancer is suspected, a biopsy of the prostate might be required. The PSA level is not necessarily a final indicator of prostate cancer. I had 3 biopsies with no positive results of cancer. I now take medication and supplements to maintain my personal levels and monitor them each year.

• Cancer of the bladder and pelvic tumors can likewise disturb the bladder and urinary recurrence.

Blood in the pee

• Hematuria or blood in the pee can be brought about by a urinary disease, kidney stones, or different causes.

•   The blood could be noticeable by the unaided eye or may be found on a pee assessment (minute hematuria).

•   For a few people, it is a manifestation of cancer of the bladder or kidney.

•   Any scene of blood in the pee ought to be researched.

Hoarseness

•   Hoarseness not brought about by respiratory disease or that keeps going longer than three to about a month ought to be assessed.

•   Hoarseness can be brought about by straightforward sensitivity or by vocal string polyps. However, it could likewise be the primary indication of cancer of the throat.

Persistent irregularities or swollen organs

•   Lumps most as often as possible speak to innocuous conditions, for example, a generous sore. A specialist ought to analyze any new bump or a protuberance that won't leave.

•   Bumps may speak to cancer or a swollen lymph organ identified with infection.

•   Lymph hubs swell from contamination and different causes and may take a long time to dry once more.

•   A knot or organ that remaining parts swelled for three to about a month ought to be assessed.

The recognizable change in a mole or a mole

• Multicolored moles that have sporadic edges or drain might be cancerous.

• More goliath moles are progressively troubling and should undergo testing, mainly if they appear to extend.

• Removing a mole is typically straightforward. You ought to have your PCP survey any suspicious mole for evacuation. The specialist will send it for assessment under a magnifying instrument for skin cancer.

Indigestion or trouble gulping

• Most individuals with constant acid reflux, as a rule, don't have severe issues.

• People who experience the ill effects of constant or enduring manifestations in spite of utilizing over-the-counter stomach settling agents may need an upper GI endoscopy.

• A condition called Barrett's throat, which can prompt cancer of the throat, can be treated with prescription and afterward checked by a specialist.

• Difficulty gulping is a typical issue, particularly in more established grown-ups, and has numerous causes.

• Swallowing issues should be examined because sustenance is continuously significant.

• Difficulty gulping solids can be seen with cancer of the throat.

Unusual vaginal draining or release

• Unusual vaginal draining or ridiculous release might be an early indication of cancer of the uterus. Ladies ought to be assessed when they have seeping after intercourse or seeping between periods.

• Bleeding that returns, that keeps going at least two days longer than anticipated, or that is heavier than expected additionally justifies medicinal assessment.

• Usually, the assessment will incorporate an endometrial biopsy, where a specialist takes a little tissue test from inside the uterus for testing.

• A Pap smear ought to be a piece of each lady's standard therapeutic consideration.

Unexpected weight reduction, night sweats, or fever

• These vague manifestations may be available with a few unique kinds of cancer. Pancreatic cancer can show up with weight reduction and no particular torment.

• Various contaminations can prompt comparable manifestations (for instance, tuberculosis).

Continued tingling in the butt-centric or genital territory

• Precancerous or cancerous states of the skin of the genital or butt-centric territories can cause constant tingling.

• Some cancers cause skin shading changes.

• Several contaminations or skin conditions (for instance, parasitic diseases or psoriasis) likewise can cause these side effects. On the off chance that tingling does not stop with over-the-counter topical drugs, your primary care physician ought to review the territory.

Nonhealing injuries

•   Sores by and large mend rapidly. On the off chance that a zone neglects to recuperate, you may have cancer and should see a specialist.

•   Nonhealing injuries in your mouth or persevering white or red fixes on your gums, tongue, or tonsils are additionally should raise concerns.

•   Some nonhealing wounds might be because of reduced flow (for instance, diabetic foot ulcers).

Headaches

•   Headaches have numerous causes (for instance, headaches, aneurysms) yet cancer is not a typical one.

•   A severe tenacious cerebral pain that feels unique concerning regular can be an indication of cancer. However, aneurysms may display similarly.

•   If your concern neglects to improve with over-the-counter meds, see a specialist quickly.

Back torment, pelvic torment, swelling, or acid reflux

•   These are typical indications of day by day life, frequently identified with nourishment admission, muscle fits or strains, yet they additionally can be seen in ovarian cancer.

•   Ovarian cancer is especially testing to treat since it is much of the time analyzed late throughout the sickness.

For further information conduct a search on the internet but check for reliable sources because there is a wealth of information. Joyce and I used the online medical library at the Kaiser Permanente patient website.

Chapter 24 – Questions to Ask Your Doctor

After being diagnosed with cancer you may find the following questions helpful in understanding the treatment process and the various services available from your insurance provider. Here are some questions to ask before you choose your cancer treatment.

Questions about Your Cancer Treatment

What are the ways to treat my type and stage of cancer?

What are the advantages and risks of those treatments?

What treatment do you recommend? Why do you think it's best for me?

When do I begin treatment?

Will I be in the hospital for treatment? If so, for how long?

What's my likelihood of recovery with this treatment?

How will you know if the treatment is working?

Would a research study be right for me?

Is Palliative care available?

Is Hospice Care available?

Questions about the various kinds of Treatment

Where will I go for treatment?

When will the treatment be given?

How long does each treatment take?

What number of treatments will I have?

Can I bring someone or a friend associate with me to my treatment?

Other Questions about side effects

What are the side effects of the treatment?

What do I need to tell you regarding the medicines I'm taking now?

Do I tell you about dietary supplements (such as vitamins, minerals, herbs, or fish oil) I'm taking?

Do I tell you about using CBD Oil or THC for pain?

Chapter 25 - Our Daily Journey with Cancer Continues

By the beginning of July in 2019 the spread of the cancer to Joyce's brain reduced her mobility and independence significantly. The whole brain radiation treatment now required a family member to take on the responsibility of Joyce's care on a daily basis. Her memory was now fading in and out. She was sometimes coherent and at other times she just drifted off to sleep.

July 28, 2019 – Day 373

4:30 AM – I awakened to find Joyce was out of bed and once again in the bathroom. I rushed out of the bed, slightly stumbled to gain my balance, as it was still dark and very little light was coming through the shutters. I walked to the master bathroom.

"What are you doing sweetie pie?" I whispered through the crack in the door opening.

"Same old shit on a new day!" Joyce answered back.

"What's your pain level?" I asked. She replied, "I'm ok no pain."

Joyce had minimum pain and for the last two and a half weeks, she also had good bowel movements. Those were the first consistent days of normal bowel movements, in over a year. During the summer break, after I reviewed her doctor's notes from her medical records for the past year, it became clear that the problems with her constipation stemmed from the pain-relieving opiates. Since Joyce was in pain and needed these drugs, she would need to take constipation medications every single day, not only when she thought she needed them. I increased her water intake and consistently gave her stool softeners, herbal laxative, and milk of magnesia twice each day.

4:55 AM

"Ok, I'm going for my walk with Tommie" I told her while walking down the hall to the front door with Tommie following behind me. Tommie and I had a daily routine of taking a walk, before I left for work.

I used these walks, as my time to have a few minutes to myself and plan my activities for the day. Tommie had become even more special, as a service dog for Joyce. He followed her everywhere she went except when I came home or took him for a walk in the mornings. Whenever I was away from home, Tommie never wakes Joyce up, for his morning walk. He never hesitated to wake me up. He will now bark when Joyce is feeling pain, and someone is not around to help. After returning from our walk, Tommie immediately went to find Joyce and laid at her feet.

While putting Tommie's leash away, I yelled out to Joyce, telling her "I'm back. Are you ready for some oatmeal?" I did not hear a response and walked back to the master bedroom. I found her leaning forward sitting on the toilet. Before I could say anything, Joyce said," I'm not asleep just hungry. Can you fix me some oatmeal and fruit?" "Sure thing, do you want one or two pack of oatmeal?", I asked her, while helping her get to her walker. "Two with four sugars (Truvia) and lots of butter", Joyce told me as she moved back in the bedroom to her favorite reclining chair, which had become her bed.

I made her oatmeal and brought it to her, along with a glass of apple juice. Going back to the kitchen and I made a pot of coffee and a bowl of fruit for her. The kitchen now smelled of fresh coffee, hazelnut creamer, strawberries, and blue berries. I re-entered our bedroom and brought Joyce her first medications for the morning.

As she finished her oatmeal, she watched me coming from the bathroom with the familiar little blue tray.

Joyce says, "Here comes the pill guy again!", she said with a smile, "I'm so lucky to have a doctor taking care of me, I love you so much". "I love you too!" I answered her softly, as I handed her one of her pills

5:45 AM

Joyce was frustrated and asked, "Why do you only give me one pill at a time?"

I told her, "Because that way I can get you to drink more water, which helps you poop everyday".

"Smart Ass! Don't say it. I know you have more degrees than Spencer on Criminal Minds", Joyce said while snickering.

I placed the fruit and a glass of juice on her TV tray and gave her a morphine and steroid pill, one at a time.

"I wish I had met you earlier!", Joyce continued, "And now I'm really tired. I need to take a nap for a little bit!"

"I love you sweetie pie", Joyce says as she closed her eyes.

I had started writing a journal and after 40 days I now had become her personal health care specialist. I noticed Joyce needed to eat something before taking her medications as this would lessen her discomfort. I was reminded once again of the importance of reading all the warnings, on each pill bottle. During the past 15 years I had never read her bottles and assumed she was competent enough to take her own medications. Afterall, she had the best doctors in the world. Over the years, I had become concerned over the amount of pills Joyce was taking. Her prescriptions had grown significantly during the past five years. I now watched my health and chose to take more herbal supplements and vitamins instead of prescription medications.

9:00 PM

I pressed the button on her recliner and covered her with her Christmas blanket, watching her closely as she fell asleep. We had not been able to sleep together or be intimate for over one year, which we both missed. I slept alone in our California King bed, while Joyce slept in a recliner next to me. I was content because she could finally get some sleep at night.

"I love you sweetie pie", Joyce said softly as she drifted off to sleep.

After taking one final look at Joyce, I got into bed. I was dead tired and needed to go to sleep. As I pulled the covers up, I remember I had forgotten to give Joyce her sleep spray. I got out of bed and grabbed the sleep support spray and lightly touched Joyce's cheek and said, "Open up and say Ahh!" With the lights still off, I squirted two sprays, hitting her cheek instead of her mouth. Joyce chuckled, "back to the firing range Marine. Hit my mouth the next time please." I turned on the light and hit my target the next time and then took five squirts for myself. "Alexa, play This is My

Promise". Alexa responded, "Playing This is My Promise, by the Temptations on Amazon Music".

The song played and I sang along with the Temptations

You're a very special part of my life

You're the one that I adore

You are my Cherie Amour

You're the one (you're the one)

I've been looking for (that I've been praying for...yes I have)

I wanna love you

(I wanna love you baby)

Better or worse

(love you for better or worse)

I wanna honor you

(I wanna honor baby)

Because you come first

(Honor because you come first)

And I will cherish you....like no other man can do This is my promise to you

(this is my promise to you)

All day long baby

(this is my promise to you)

There will never be another you

You would make my heart complete

(make your little heart complete)

And I supply your every need (OOOOHHH)

I wanna know will you marry me oh oh oh oh oh

I wanna care for you (I wanna care you baby)

In sickness and health (whether in sickness or health)

And I promise baby (and I promise you baby)

There will be no one else.....(love you and nobody else)

I'll even die for you (don't you know I will die for you

And to thine ownself....I'll be true (this is my promise to you)

And this is my promise to you

(this is my promise to you)

This is my promise baby

Every night I told Alexa to play this song, which would always put us both to sleep. Sixteen years ago, on February 14, 2003 Joyce fell in love with a singing Karaoke DJ when I sang "I'll Make Love to You by Boyz 2 Men." She fell in love once, again each night, hoping to wake up the next morning and have just one more day with me. Her love for me gave her the will to live. The thought of her love allowed me to fall asleep until my alarm went off at 5 AM.

Chapter 26 – Compassionate Care is Possible

Palliative care (pronounced pal-lee-uh-tiv) is a specialized medical aid for people living with a significant illness. This type of care concentrates on relieving the symptoms and stress from a life- threatening illness. The goal is to boost the quality of life for each patient and therefore the family.

Both Palliative care and Hospice Care give comfort. However, palliative care should begin at the same time treatment begins. Hospice care should begin once curative treatment of an illness has stopped and when it's clear the patient does not wish to prolong their life.

Hospice care is analogous to palliative care, however there are vital variations. Hospice patients should meet Medicare's eligibility requirements; palliative care patients do not need to meet an equivalent requirement.

The definition of Hospice Care is compassionate comfort care, for people facing a terminal illness, with a prognosis of six months or less to live. Palliative Care is also compassionate comfort car, which gives relief from the symptoms and physical and/or mental stress of a life-limiting illness. The target of each is pain and symptom relief. In retrospect, we should have selected Palliative Care at the beginning of Joyce's diagnosis, of stage 4 terminal cancer.

The American Society of Clinical medicine defines the characteristics of a patient receiving palliative care as follows:

☐ The patient has restricted ability to care for themself.

☐ The patient has received curative treatment and isn't taking advantage of it any longer.

☐ The patient doesn't qualify for a limited degree acceptable medical trial.

☐ There is no proof that more treatment would be effective.

Hospice eligibility needs two physicians to certify that the patient has but six months to live, if the illness follows its natural course. Palliative care begins at the discretion of the doctor and patient at any time, at any stage of unwellness, terminal or not.

Some organizations can deliver both hospice and palliative care. They address physical, emotional and non-secular pain, together with such common worries as loss of independence, the well-being of the family and the feeling of being a burden.

Hospice care expenses are paid, one hundred percent, by your health care insurance. By comparison, palliative care costs —from health care provider visits,to prescription charges—can vary. Hospice care is delivered at your home or in home-like hospice residences, nursing homes, aided living facilities, veterans' facilities, hospitals and alternative facilities. Palliative care groups generally select a primary hospital. Talk to your family and your doctor regarding your goals of care and whether or not Palliative Care and/or Hospice Care may improve your quality of life.

We were fortunate to have a health care provider, which provided both palliative and hospice care. Because of my research and analysis of our health care plans I was able to contact a social worker, who had been assigned to Joyce's oncology department. I was able to secure a doctor's order for palliative and hospice care in September of 2019. A palliative care nurse visited our home to conduct an initial assessment, which was quite thorough in determining the exact pain relief care Joyce needed. Next, a social worker sat down with us to discuss other needs and explained the funding source for different types of care as we moved forward.

We found out that a palliative team is more than just a nurse. It is a complete team of medical professionals including a doctor, physical therapist, nurse, home health aides, and a social worker. This reduces the amount of *out of pocket* expenses for private home health care services, which start at a cost of $25 an hour.

The only issue for us, was our health care provider required all dogs must be locked up. This was a medical protocol requirement, because of past incidents of aggressive animals in the home. This rule is to protect the health care workers. Our little dog Tommie was a pain in the butt and did not want to be away from Joyce. As a result, I had to purchase a dog cage and a non-shock dog collar. But that still didn't work, because Tommie was so protective of Joyce. He would bark like crazy, unless he was lying right at her feet. I had to train Tommie to change his habits. I found a compromise by simply putting him on a leash, whenever health care personnel were present. After one week, Tommie adapted to his new rules.

Chapter 27 - The Counter Offensive

During my summer vacations, in 2018 and 2019, I sat in our bedroom, most days, watching Joyce to make sure she was comfortable. Her pain had become manageable, but the onset of any new treatment brought about changes in our search to end her constipation. She wanted to stop taking Milk of Magnesia and that resulted in the return of her constipation. Once again, we had to continue with the established routine. Between immunotherapy and radiation treatments, Joyce was prescribed a dexamethasone steroid. It took 16 days to get off that steroid, and it caused an increase in her use of Norco, which was another opiate.

On August 1, 2019, Joyce began her third try at chemotherapy. This time the dosage was much stronger. Her treatments began with two weeks on and one week off. She had just been through radiation, which made her very tired and lethargic. She was starting to sleep more and more each day. Her appetite decreased sharply. She lost her appetite for her favorite breakfast of cinnamon & spice oatmeal with fruit. She was now totally unaware of her bowel movement accidents. She had little control over her bladder even though she didn't like to wear adult diapers, and wanted to get back to wearing her regular underwear. Her adult diapers were now giving her a rash and starting to itch. She had an accident and then knew her regular underwear were a thing of the past. She needed help getting in and out of her lounge chair. It helped that the recliner was fully motorized and lifted her up, making it easier to get her out of it. She needed assistance going to the bathroom and taking a shower on a daily basis. Her communication skills had decreased, and she was highly fatigued. The chemo brought back the awful taste of food and she lost her appetite, once again. Her weight was deceiving because of the excess water in her left leg. She now required the full support of care givers to do the minimal functions of life. I could not take care of her myself, because I had to continue working. Retirement was no longer possible, especially now because of Joyce's condition. I now needed to work to prepare for the loss in monthly income, when Joyce would pass away.

August 11, 2019 was the 386th day after her diagnosis with stage four cancer. The original cancer had spread throughout her lymph nodes and into her brain. This was a secondary malignant growth. Joyce had traveled back and forth to hospital over 130 times, for three different treatments, including chemotherapy, immunotherapy, and radiation to the pelvic area lymph nodes and even whole brain radiation treatments.

Her brief moments of depression were increasing in frequency each week. She was growing weary of her personal, physical and mental limitations. She became argumentative with her care givers and family. This was because she realized her mental capabilities were not the same. She was tired of going to the emergency room and waiting for hours just to find out that little help was available. She was tired of all of the shots and pain pills every day and wanted to feel normal once again. I knew things would only get worse in the near future.

11:00 AM, August 21, 2019

As I was driving to work that morning, I was concerned about the swelling and redness in Joyce's left leg. It was clear to me that her medication, might be stopping her blood clots from increasing, but it was not relieving the pain and redness in her leg. I contacted the Palliative Care hotline and left a message that I needed to speak with the doctor. When I returned home from work, I received a call from the doctor, and we agreed to put her back on a previous medication, which had worked after her visit to an emergency room, just three weeks ago.

6:20 AM August 22, 2019 (Day 398)

As I was taking a shower and getting dressed for work, I heard Alexa announce, "There is motion at the Jordan front driveway." After a few seconds, Alexa continued, "There is motion at the Jordan front door". I looked at Joyce and said to our Echo device, "Alexa show the front driveway!" Alexa displayed the driveway on the Echo Show screen. I recognized the car in the driveway belonging to Christina.

Christina and Nick had arrived to take over caring for Joyce, and to take her to her next chemo treatment that day. Nick was Christina's son and Joyce's grandson. Joyce took custody of Nick when he was only two years old, he was more like a son to her than a grandson.

As I opened the master bedroom door, Christina looked in and said, "Good morning sunshine" to her mother.

I reviewed Joyce's daily routine, with Christina and asked her to pick up her mother's new prescription. We jointly maintained a journal and communicated frequently, during the day to ensure that Joyce was as comfortable as possible. Unlike a year ago, I now felt more comfortable with Christina taking care of her mother. We had our ups and downs (wrecking the car and lying), but now she was given the opportunity to make up for her past mistakes. My no non-sense military style forced Christina to be more responsible. She enrolled in school to finally finish her high school diploma, at a local adult education school.

Christiana announced to Joyce, "Mom, I'm enrolled in school to get my diploma."

Joyce's eyes began to water, as she looked up at Christy and said, "Finish what you start! That will make me very proud of you."

I gathered my bags and kissed Joyce goodbye and told her, "I've got to go. Love you."

As I closed the door, I heard sounds of Christina and Joyce laughing together about something. That sound of laughter was a moment to treasure, which set my mind at ease. Joyce began sleeping more and more each day. Was it the medications she was taking? Or was this a sign of things getting worse?

Friday, August 23, 2019 (Day 399)

The palliative nurse called to schedule an appointment with Joyce for later that morning. The social worker also scheduled a visitation for 3 PM, that same afternoon. I arrived home just as the social worker was finishing up. Joyce said that the nurse had scheduled a blood test, with an outside provider, who would call before leaving to come to our house. I was upset because I was not informed of this additional visitation. I was confused when Christina told me that Joyce had answered a phone call, but she was unclear what the call was for.

3:45 PM

Joyce told me, "I am getting my blood drawn and she will call before leaving Riverside."

5:30 PM

I said, "This doesn't make sense. Who is coming? Joyce told me, "they will call before coming!"

I then decided to verify this appointment by calling the nurse, who confirmed the order for the blood test, but could not tell me who and when?"

Joyce became very upset that I didn't understand, and that I believed something was wrong. I called Christy to ask her about the appointment, but she could not verify it and suggested I look at the caller ID. I retrieved the phone number, and after calling it back, I confirmed the approximate time of the appointment to be around 6:30 PM.

7:15 PM.

Erica called later to confirmed her approximate arrival time at 7:45 PM. She arrived at 7:50 PM and drew Joyce's blood. I was very concerned about health care providers calling to make appointments through Joyce. In my opinion Joyce was no longer capable of taking these calls until her mental state improved. Appointments made after 8 PM, on a Friday evening, were unacceptable to me. The blood test was already overdue and could have been taken on Saturday morning. On the bright side it was important for me to learn about another service, which was provided by our palliative care team. I wondered if Joyce's pre-chemo blood could be drawn as well and made a note to speak with the doctor. The blood test was the CEA test, which for some reason was still not being released, and visible on our medical website. I was upset because I had to send an email in order to get this test result. I felt this was an unnecessary additional step for us to go through at this stage in our cancer battle.

August 29, 2019 (Day 406)

Christy and Nick took Joyce to her next chemo treatment. After checking our medical provider's website, I told Joyce that her CEA results were at 395. This was a decrease of nearly 40%, indicating the chemo treatment was working to decrease the cancer proteins spreading throughout her body. Upon their return home, Christy told me the oncologist told her there was a slight decrease in the size of some of Joyce's tumors, but not the one in her pancreas. Christy told me the doctor's statements seemed to give her mother a false sense of hope.

As an in-home care support person, Christy recognized the signs of death her mother was exhibiting on a daily basis. Christy shared this information with me, before she left for her home that day. She also told me, "it's only going to get worse!" "The doctor said to get a donut pillow for Joyce and to try and get her back into bed, to sleep at night." "You need to buy a bedside commode," Christy told me.

"What the hell is that?", I asked myself." I did a Google search and found out it is an adult portable potty. I then ordered additional hand grips for the shower and bathroom walls to make it safer for Joyce. The new chemo was taking its toll on Joyce, as she now needed assistance to get back and forth from the toilet. She had no problem going to sleep that night. She slept throughout the night, for the first time, in over a year. I reminded her that I would call around noon the next day.

August 30, 2019

Joyce slept throughout the night once again. It had been over a year since we shared the same bed. I woke up many times, each night, to see if Joyce was asleep in her recliner. I was pleased to see she was still resting. It was now 4:30 AM, so I got up and followed my daily routine of walking Tommie. I felt safe because of our new Ring App on my phone which allowed me to watch Joyce, as she slept quietly. After my walk and checking on Joyce, I got in the shower and thought about work. I was already dressed when Christy and Nick arrived at 6:35 AM. I woke Joyce to take her to the bathroom. She was being stubborn and wanted to walk by herself. Joyce was losing strength, on a daily basis, and needed assistance to get out of her recliner and into her walker. With me leading the way, she slowly took six steps. All of a sudden she stopped, closing her eyes, losing her balance and fell backwards to the floor on her butt, then her back, hitting her head on the carpeted floor.

I yelled, "CHRISTY! I need your help!" We checked Joyce's head for wounds or bleeding and found no noticeable damage. We got her back into her walker and moved her safely to the bathroom. Once again, we checked her head. By this time, it was almost 7 AM and I needed to leave for work. As I was backing out of the garage, I thought back to a conversation with one of my co-workers, who was dealing with a similar situation. Yesterday she told me, how her husband fell and broke his pelvic bone right before a scheduled out-patient surgery. This had been Joyce's first fall.

I made a call to the Palliative Care office to report Joyce's fall, letting them know what had happened and asked for recommendations. The nurse deemed the incident as not requiring immediate attention, because of her regularly scheduled visit in a few hours. The palliative care nurse was scheduled to arrive that morning between 8:30-9:30. After examining Joyce, she advised us that in the future, if she fell and hit her head, we should immediately take her to the emergency room. Upon hearing the nurses' comments Joyce said, "I'm tired of that place!" I nodded my head in agreement.

Joyce had been to the emergency room numerous times. After this fall, I would now walk closely behind her to ensure that another fall did not take place. Whenever she had to go to the bathroom, I would place my hands on her hips, she turned and said, "Oh honey keep your hands Right Thur!", as she took each step forward slowly pushing her walker. I thought to myself these walks would need to end soon, because my arm was still hurting, from lifting her off the floor this morning.

My weekends would never be the same. I was still working fulltime. Labor Day weekend ended three days of care giving tasks for me. I had taken over full responsibility, to ensure the bills were paid, the checkbook was balanced, grocery shopping was completed, and all household chores, including the laundry was done. One year ago, those tasks were done jointly by both of us. I love her dearly, but this fight with cancer was taking its toll on me, both physically, emotionally and mentally. Every day, during the week I had to rely on non-productive, undependable and irresponsible stepchildren to care for Joyce, so I could continue working, which was still a financial necessity.

Chapter 28 – Quantity Versus Quality of Life

In August of 2019, we asked her oncologist for a referral to Palliative care services. These services were designed for people who have a serious advanced health condition or a life-threatening illness. In retrospect, I felt that we should have started Joyce on these services, after her initial diagnosis, in August of 2018, but Joyce wanted to remain at home and have family members take care of her. This was a mistake, as we had assumed this care meant she would be taken to a health care facility. We both did not fully understand how these additional services and this care could have helped improve our quality of life.

In September of 2019, Joyce's oncologist told us that we would need to make a decision about quantity versus quality of life. When Joyce first heard her diagnosis, of stage four cancer, her immediate thought was about her remaining quantity of life. Her quantity of life referred to how many days she had left to live. She thought to herself, "How many days would I have left to spend with my loving husband and family?" For Joyce, this really meant how many Christmas Eves were left in her lifetime. But at some point, this quantity of life would not mean a quality of life. She dealt with her pain in order to have more time to plan her last Christmas Eve, in 2018. She hid the amount of pain she was experiencing, even from me. Our quantity of life was preoccupied with trips back and forth to medical facilities. There was very little quality of life experienced at this time.

Before Joyce's cancer diagnosis, our quality of life was funded by both of our incomes. After her diagnosis this quality of life diminished every month and our credit card balances slowly began to creep up. While taking care of Joyce, I was also supporting a stepdaughter and step-grandson, who haven't had decent jobs for the past several years and were primarily living off of us. We supplied them with money for gas, car repairs, and even cell phone service so Joyce would be able to have daily contact with them. During our marriage we paid their housing expenses, for several years. I never approved of this situation and continually explained to Joyce how this was spoiling these irresponsible adult children. I could have retired by then, if it had not been for spending thousands of dollars supporting these grown adults. Over the years this translated into thousands of dollars in credit card debt. We lost our big two-story home in 2009, after the economic collapse of 2007. I then insisted we move to a 55+ community, so that none of our adult children could ever live with us again. I began saving extra money each month into a "keep them away" account. But finally, I happily closed the "Bank of Jordan, in 2017." I simply could not continue the hemorrhaging of money to support adults who refused to grow up. However, I continued to honor the promise I made to Joyce's mother, not to interfere with her spirit of Christmas.

During our last years together, before her cancer diagnosis, I just chose to work more and be at home less often. This was my way of coping with the stepchildren. Our battle with cancer would just aggravate this situation, because now I would have to continue to pay Joyce's children each week, just to care for their own mother and grandmother. I was working in excess of 53 hours every week, which included 13-hour days on Tuesday through Thursday, teaching adult education and not returning home after 8:30 at night. I just needed to manage things until March of 2020, when I was scheduled to receive my Social Security Administration (SSA) benefits. I had planned to stop teaching those night school classes, when those payments began.

Whenever a cancer patient makes a decision for the quantity of life over the quality of life, they do not realize the impact this decision will have on their families. I thought back to a comment made by Joyce's oncologist after received the results of her MRI, indicating that the cancer had spread to her brain. She told Joyce, "You will be on chemo treatments for the rest of your life!" The choice of choosing a quantity of life will require long term care, by either non-working family members or home health care personnel. Residential home health care personnel are not licensed medical personnel. I was forced to use our non-working adult children as the less expensive option.

During the past year Joyce had received two different types of chemotherapy and radiation treatments, to her lymph nodes in her abdomen and her entire brain. Each trip to the doctor required someone to be with her for 4-5 hours each treatment. We were lucky to have a cancer policy in force. This policy provided additional funds to help with every chemo and radiation visit. Later, when Joyce decided not to receive chemo the additional funds stopped, which created a huge financial deficit each and every week.

In August of 2019, Joyce started a more aggressive chemo treatment, which required her to receive treatments for two weeks on and then one week off. She received treatments on August 1st, 8th, 22nd, and 29th. She was scheduled for an office appointment on September 5, 2019. She was now on 60 mg dosage of morphine every day just to keep her free of pain, but the chemo treatments this time around ruined her taste buds and appetite. She was taking laxatives and Milk of Magnesia every day. She loved strawberries and blueberries with cinnamon oatmeal every morning for breakfast. Her food intake had drastically decreased, to simple mouthfuls of food. Joyce weighed 216 lbs. over a year ago and now her weigh was 160 lbs. and dropping. For the first time in our marriage Joyce weighed less than I did.

Her current health and battle with cancer, also brought about complications with her dental care. Joyce had a nagging toothache and needed a tooth to be pulled but the dentist would not extract the tooth because of all the blood thinners she was on. The dentist also believed the chemo treatments would prevent the wound from healing properly. Joyce's legs continued to swell, which now required daily shots to keep the swelling in her left leg under control. She was no longer diabetic, but now had to receive other injections because of her other health issues. She could no longer use her walker and those of us caring for her had to lift her from her recliner to the bedside commode. She was now sleeping long periods throughout the day. On September 4, I contacted the palliative nurse and requested a feeding tube, because of her lack of food intake.

When I returned home from work that day, I gave Joyce her evening shot and bedtime pills and then helped her out of her recliner to the bedside commode. She was weak and extremely tired. I asked her about her pain level, and she responded by looking up at me and saying, "I'm done with this shit! I don't want to live like this anymore." I said, "I understand baby!" We then discussed stopping chemo treatments and made a decision to contact her oncologist asking her for a referral, assigning Joyce to Hospice Care. After she fell asleep, I went to my computer and sent an email to the oncologist requesting the medical referral.

Chapter 29 - The Final Battle - Hospice Care

Joyce was in pain daily, throughout her battle with cancer. She was taking a lot of opioids, which unfortunately, had a major side effect of constipation. But the key information, she was never told, was that her daily treatment for constipation would need to continue for the rest of her life.

It had been over a year and I was desperately seeking a solution for Joyce's pain. I did not work during the summer, because I was a teacher. So, this summer while caring for Joyce I began to collect observational data. I used my mathematical reasoning skills to chart her pain, her food intake, and her bowel movements. I started working with her doctors to try and eliminate her nagging pain and discomfort.

I took charge of all interactions with her doctor, regarding her medications needed for pain management. I sent a final email to her oncologist requesting more antibiotics for Joyce's leg before hospice took over her care. The Hospice Care center called me to set-up an appointment for Monday September 9, 2019. I was there for the first nurse visit. Joyce officially began receiving hospice care on the 10th of September.

Hospice care is designed for people in their final stage of life, when the patient no longer wants to prolong their life. Hospice is paid by Medi-care. Hospice Care provided a complete team of medical personnel. There would be no more trips to pick-up prescriptions or emergency trips to the hospital. Part of our hospice agreement was we would no longer have to call 911. They provided me with a number I could call 24/7, so all future medical services would be provided at home. This was a dramatic improvement to our quality of life.

During her hospice care Joyce received two visits a week from an assigned nurse, two visits a week from a bedside nurse for bathing, weekly visits from a social worker, a chaplain, a physical therapist, and weekly visits from a dedicated doctor. Her hospice care doctor had previously been assigned as her palliative care doctor. The assigned hospice travel nurse lived only three blocks from us, and was on call 24 hours a day. Everything was done from the comfort of our home, including blood tests and prescription refills. Hospice provided everything, even medical items to make her comfortable. I had already purchased many of the items that hospice would have provided. I wish we had been told about Hospice Care earlier. Joyce had been off of chemo treatments for two weeks when her nagging tooth finally fell out on its own.

By September 12, our home had been transformed into a virtual hospital, with a hospital bed, body lifter and harness, oxygen tanks, and a box of medications to keep Joyce comfortable, and out of pain. Medical equipment was spread throughout the house.

It has been over one year since Joyce's cancer diagnosis and she was now unable to walk to the bathroom on her own. Her lack of balance made it difficult for anyone to move her by themselves. Her bedside nurse requested she be placed in the hospital bed, which would make it easier to give her a sponge bath. Joyce continued to fight and refused to go potty in her adult diapers. She had a couple of falls because of this and I was determined to get her out of her recliner, so I began developing a strategy to get her into that damn hospital bed. Her bedside commode was placed right next to her recliner, in the corner of our master bedroom. Diapers, sanitary latex gloves, and baby wipes were positioned close by for her daily care. Pads were placed under the bedside commode in case she had an accident.

Joyce had now been on Hospice Care for nearly three weeks. Her pain level was practically zero, due to the additional comfort medications. She was unable to swallow pills, even the smallest ones, and now required liquid forms of her medications.

Friday, October 11, 2019 was the beginning of another weekend of caring for Joyce by myself. I would have little time for anything else. I brought her meals and made sure she took her medications. I would move her to the bedside commode and then clean her with the disposable wipes and changed her clothing if necessary. Joyce was very agitated during that weekend. She was trying to write notes in her journal, but when I looked at them, I could not read her writing.

My quality of life did not exist. The palliative care nurse suggested that I take a five-day sabbatical, but I did not want to leave Joyce. I was not sleeping for more than a couple of hours each night.

On Sunday October 13, of 2019, Joyce finally fell asleep around 11 PM. I was exhausted and had to return to work the next morning. I drifted off to sleep by telling, "Alexa, play This is My Promise!" Alexa responded, "Playing This is My Promise by the Temptations on Amazon Music, starting now!" After taking four squirts of my sleep support spray, I finally fell asleep while listening to the music.

I was awakened by the noise of the recliner moving upward.

Joyce was trying to get up. I asked, "What are you doing?" She responded, "I got to go now." I told her, "Ok Wait a minute!" I quickly got out of bed and helped her to the bedside commode. Joyce had to go really bad and couldn't hold it. I heard a loud splash into the bucket. Joyce sighed and I looked for a fresh diaper and baby-wipes to clean her with and placed them on the bed. I looked at the clock and noticed that it was now 2:30 in the morning. I was half asleep when I walked to the kitchen for a drink of water, before returning to the bedroom.

When I returned, I saw something dripping on the pad beneath Joyce. As I moved closer, I saw the color of the puddle, below the commode, was fresh red blood. There was a lot more blood around the top of the commode seat, where Joyce was sitting. I checked further around the commode to see where the blood was coming from and finally realized it was coming from Joyce. I didn't want to upset or alarm her, so I grabbed the phone and called our Hospice Care center to request that a nurse come out right away.

I explained to the nurse that there was a massive amount of blood coming from Joyce's rectum. She wanted to get back into her recliner, but I told her to stay put, because I needed to clean up the mess. I carefully cleaned her, then helped her stand, so I could see the extent of the bleeding. When I checked the commode, I found a pool of blood and diarrhea. After cleaning her, I placed her back into her recliner. I kept the soiled materials in order to show them to the nurse. I was scared because I knew this was not normal or good. Joyce was having internal bleeding. Upon arrival the nurse confirmed my fears and told me that things may get worse and this was another reason we needed to get her into the hospital bed and for her to use diapers. I sent a message to my school secretary and told her I was taking the day off. I was fortunate to have a good job and the support of co-workers, which allowed me to take all the time I needed to care for Joyce.

After a discussion with our family, we moved her hospital bed into the living room to provide better access for medical personnel, and to give me some privacy in the bedroom, so I could finally get a good night's sleep. Our master bedroom had been a hospital room for the past five months. I would now be able to sleep at night, during the week and have family members take care of her. I asked for the support of her family. I knew Joyce did not have much time left. I put aside my differences with her sister and allowed close friends to visit during her final days.

Joyce's health conditions rapidly deteriorated during that next week. She would not eat, and her blood pressure started to fall. The last time she spoke was on Tuesday, October 15, 2019. She told her daughter, "People think that just because I'm sick I don't know I gotta pee!" Joyce grabbed her daughter's shirt, with all her might and yelled," I'm telling you that I gotta pee right now!

The Joyce our family knew and loved left this earth during the third week in October. She passed away at home surrounded by her loving husband and family at 4:18 PM, on October 21, 2019. Her memorial service was held at Miller Jones Mortuary, on November 11, 2019 and she was buried at the Riverside National Memorial Cemetery on November 12, 2019.

Chapter 30 – Lessons Learned

As a U. S. Marine Officer, I had been accustomed in reviewing lessons learned, from after-action reports, from numerous operational exercises. Marine Officers are trained to reflect on previous actions taken, so that we could make improvements and not repeat past mistakes. At Annapolis, the incoming Midshipmen are required to read the History of Naval Sea Power, and review past naval battles and strategies, during armed conflicts. As an artillery and logistics officer, I would review and develop new strategies that would save lives during the 1st Gulf War in Iraq and Kuwait. Facing Death together is more about reflections and lessons learned during our battle with stage 4 cancer.

Reflective Thoughts

I have learned, throughout my lifetime, that this reflective process is necessary to make self-improvements. It took me years to finally realize and look forward to learning new things each and every day. Every day brings an opportunity to learn something new and to share that knowledge in order to help others. This book was about facing death together, with my loving wife, Joyce. This was a real-life experience that allowed me to reflect back on critical mistakes, regarding our personal affairs. The following reflections are in no particular order of occurrence.

Mobility Equipment for Quality of Life

During the two months before receiving the news of stage four cancer, Joyce had difficulty in walking and dealt with the constipation issues. The cancer had started to impact her ability to walk normally and her vision. I ordered a four-prong walking cane for her to use inside the house. Later I purchased a walker with wheels and also a foldable wheelchair, to assist us during hospital visits. When Joyce hurt her left leg, by simply getting up from the toilet, early in April of 2018, I purchased handicap toilet seats with handlebars and non-slip pads to place in the showers and bathtubs. The traditional shower heads were replaced with dual shower heads and a handheld sprayer.

Mobility aids are devices designed to assist people who have problems moving around. This gives them greater freedom and independence. Typically, people who have cancer are at an increased risk of falling. These devices provide several benefits to users, including more independence, reduced pain, and increased confidence and self-esteem. A range of mobility devices are available to meet an individual's physical needs. I made the following purchases from Amazon.com, my favorite store.

- Quad Walking Canes

- Walker with wheels

- Drive Portable Wheelchair

- Replacement parts (walker knobs & boots for canes)

- ☐ Elevated leg cushions

- ☐ Emergency Life Alert Device

- ☐ Handicap Toilet seats

- ☐ Toilet seat cushions

- ☐ Lifting Safety Belt

- ☐ Bedside Commode

- ☐ Hand Grip Shower Handles

- ☐ Safety Handgrips for bathroom

- ☐ Shower safety non-slip floor mats

Home Security Enhancements

Home security became a major concern when Joyce started to receive palliative care visitations. She was primarily living in the master bedroom, far away from the front door. Today there are several different types of audio/video features, which can provide remote access via a mobile device app. I purchased the Ring doorbell system and floodlights for the outside of our house to reinforce my security concerns. Later I learned how to integrate them, using the Alexa Echo Show and Alexa Skills. I also needed to purchase a Wi-Fi extender, which would boost the signal throughout our property. I could now leave the house, for work ,or to run errands, and have complete peace of mind. I was now able to remotely monitor and see Joyce when I was not at home.

Family Volunteers are a Necessary Evil

Joyce's whole brain radiation treatment took a toll on her ability to move around on her own. It became necessary for someone to be with her 24 hours a day. Our American Fidelity Cancer policy provided limited financial resources to assist with the purchase of mobility and security equipment. I realized that providing 24-hour care for Joyce presented financial challenges. Family would need to volunteer, during this time. If everyone had been working and had stable jobs, then maybe they could contribute financially for outside help.

I remembered my tour of duty in Japan and the absence of old folk homes. The Japanese culture required the eldest child to live at home and care for aging parents. In contrast, it is unfortunate that most elderly Americans have family members who expect to be paid to assist in caring for their aging parents. Sometimes a patient, who is fighting cancer, will try to stay alive for the sake of those dear to them. This desire for a quantity of life sometimes causes more harm than good.

Necessary Insurance Products

There is a big difference in medical documentation between palliative and hospice care. A person's age is a major factor when making a decision about health and life insurance products. Joyce and I had a joint-survivorship policy that we had been paying on for 15 years, only to have it automatically cancelled when Joyce turned 70 years old. One of the many reasons I became a teacher was because of the many benefits it provided, especially the health care and life insurance policies.

More importantly I wanted to make sure that in the event of my death Joyce would have sufficient funds to continue without me. We also purchased a sufficient amount of insurance on Joyce, to provide a financial relief fund for both of us. In other words, I would receive just enough money to eliminate any debt. Because

Joyce was older, we purchased enough insurance to pay off our debts and have sufficient reserves, which would allow her to continue in our current lifestyle, in case of my death. I thought that Joyce would outlive me.

Read Before Signing

One of the lessons I learned was failing to read documents completely. Every insurance contract must be read thoroughly. You need to have a complete knowledge of all benefits and how to file a claim. I found it very important to begin and maintain a journal of all communications and actions taken, with each insurance provider. I also discovered that it was important to know how to register a complaint, in order to help expedite service and claims.

A Good Habit of Saving

A good insurance plan must be preceded by a habit of saving money. We learned during our lifetime that Murphy's Law is alive and well. When we married, we started saving a portion of our income by opening savings accounts, in our credit union. We continued saving until we had saved at least six months of fixed living expenses. After that I began having money deducted from my paycheck and deposited into an 403(b)-investment account. This habit of savings continued throughout the years of our marriage, and allowed our life together to prosper. We went from no credit and no money to good credit and a savings account, in a matter of years. Tough times came when the economy took a nose- dive in 2007. Our years of saving and understanding the credit protocols helped to eliminate our debt and to rebuild our credit, within seven years.

Never Cancel Insurance to Eliminate Murphy's Law

The purpose of insurance is to obtain risk protection in case of a loss of property or income. I recommend if you purchase a life insurance policy, you must read it thoroughly, before finalizing your purchase. Do the math to determine the amount of insurance coverage you can afford or not afford. Never cancel your insurance, when times get tough. You should make other cutbacks and adjust your budget during tough times. It is highly recommended that you purchase life insurance as early as possible, while you are healthy and young. There should be a balance between both whole life and term insurance plans.

We had purchased multiple policies from four different insurance companies. Both of the major policies had a terminal illness rider. Because I was a teacher, and was still working, Joyce was not eligible for VA assistance programs. Our cancer policy provided supplemental payments for chemo treatments, pain medications, and out-patient surgical expenses. The American General Life policy finally paid the terminal illness benefit to Joyce, two months after we filed a claim. It was necessary to obtain a doctor's statement and her complete medical records for the past two years in order to expedite payment of the benefit.

When I filed for the same terminal illness benefit with American Fidelity, they denied my claim. The reason was that my policy stated that the minimum benefit payable was $10,000. Because Joyce's policy had a face value of only $15,000 dollars the stated 50% benefit of $7,500 would not be paid. After I complained, through my employer's benefit support agency, American Fidelity (AF) decided to make an exception, to the original policy, and paid a benefit of 50% of the policy's face value, since the current version of the same policy corrected this issue. AF remains flawless in their customer support. It took two months to receive the proceeds of $7,500.

Create and Maintain a Living Trust

It was very important for us to have taken the time to develop and execute a Living Trust. The Trust provided all the necessary Powers of Attorney for finances and medical issues. However, in retrospect it should have been created by an attorney. We had originally created the trust in 2009 and then revised it in 2017, after buying a new home. Since that time, the state and federal agencies had published two important insurance policy laws, changing Trust documents. The first is an Advance Health Directive and the other is a HIPPA form. So, although there maybe inexpensive software available, I recommend you should still have a legal professional review the provisions of a Living Trust, as laws do change.

In this chapter I have shared some of my most important reflections about lessons I learned while facing this death experience. I hope that the information in this book and the sharing of our story will help someone while Facing Death Together.

List of Key Medical and Insurance Terms

Accelerated Benefit Rider
Adenocarcinoma right lung upper lobe
Arbitration
Cancer Policy
Cancer metastatic to Brain
Cancer metastatic to Lymph Node Adenocarcinoma
Chemotherapy
Complete Blood Count (CBC Differential)
Chronic Obstructive Pulmonary Disease (COPD)
Diabetes Type 2
Diagnosis
Diverticulosis of Colon
Edema (Swelling of Legs)
Essential Hypertension
Kaiser FACE Report
Family History of Melanoma (Malignant tumor)
History of Anal Cancer
History of Basal Cell Skin Cancer
Hospice Care
Hyperlipidemia (High Blood Fats)
Incidental finding of mass in the adrenal gland
Infusion
Immunotherapy
Itemized Bill
In Home Health Support

Long Term Care
Lung Cancer Metastatic to unspecified site
Lymph Nodes
Malignant tumor
Metastatic
Osteoporosis (significant thinning of the bone)
Palliative Care
Radiation therapy
Release of Medical Records
Saline Solution
Surgical units
Terminal Illness Rider
Tumor
Unremarkable
Visit Summary
Vulvar Intraepithelial Neoplasia 3

Suggested Resources

Cancer.gov (2019). *Cancer treatment types.* Retrieved from *https://www.cancer.gov/about-cancer/treatment/types/*

Loveliveson.com (2019). *Signs of death.* Retrieved from *https://www.loveliveson.com/signs-of-death/*

Miller-Jones.com (2019). *Plan ahead.* Retrieved from https://www.miller-jones.com/plan-ahead/advance-directives

Vitas.com (2019). *Hospice and Palliative care.* Retrieved fromhttps://www.vitas.com/hospice-and-palliative-care-basics/about-palliative-care/hospice-vs-palliative-care-whats-the-difference

Webmd.com (2019). *What is ultrasound.* Retrieved from https://www.webmd.com/a-to-z-guides/what-is-an-ultrasound

Iwmf.com (2016). *CBC results explained.* Retrieved from https://www.iwmf.com/sites/default/files/docs/bloodcharts_cbc(1).pdf

Other Important Links

Chemotherapy and You: Support for People with Cancer
Celebration of Life Ideas | Beach Theme
Radiation Therapy and You: Support for People with Cancer

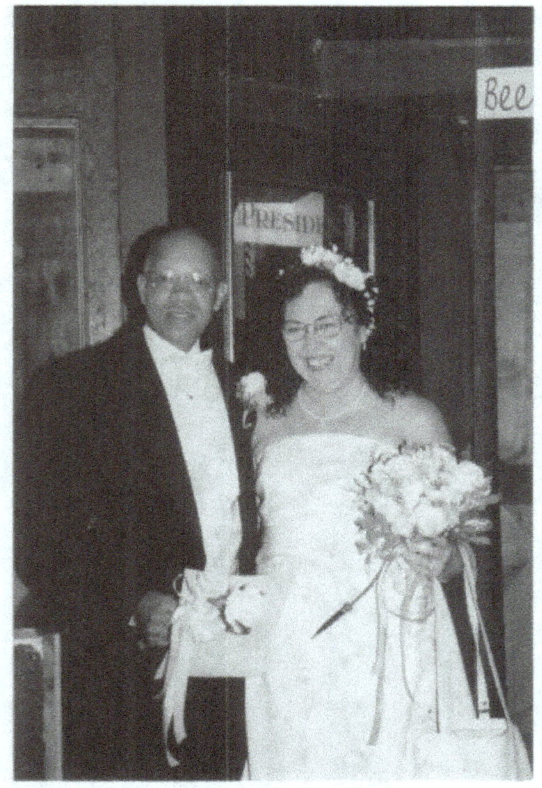

Jordan and Joyce Smith – Wedding Reception – Sept 2003

About the Author

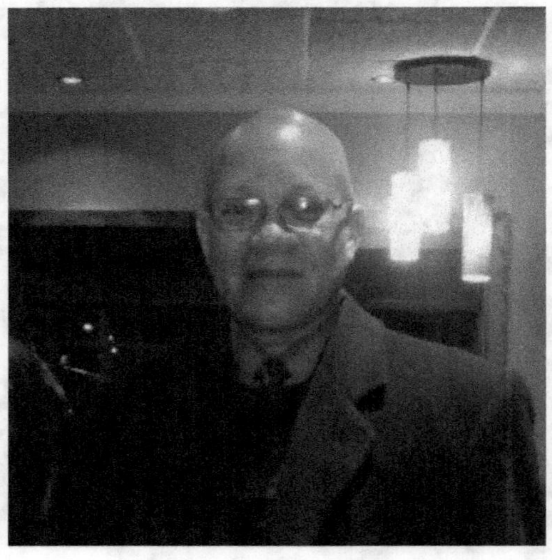

Jordan B. Smith Jr. Ed. D.

I am a mathematician, teacher, author, producer, and public speaker who was born and grew up in St. Louis, Missouri where I attended Lexington Grade School (K-8) and graduated from Christian Brothers College Military Institute in Clayton, Missouri. I left my hometown in 1972 to attend the United States Naval Academy where I became the first African American to be chosen as the Color Company Commander in 1976. I served 20 years in the U. S. Marine Corps and I am a veteran of the first Gulf War (1990-1991). I am a public high school teacher in Southern California. I have conducted multiple presentations for the California Mathematics Council (CMC), California Association of the Gifted (CAG), and California Continuation Education Association (CCEA) during the past four years. I was scheduled to speak at the National Council of Supervisors of Mathematics (NCSM) in April 2020 reporting upon research and instructional practices making make fun to learn.

I have been a member of Visitation Committees for the Accrediting Commission for Schools, Western Association of Schools and Colleges (ACS WASC) since 2015 and a chairperson since 2019. I was selected in 2019 as a Model School Field Expert for the California Department of Education in 2019 for alternative schools. I am the author of Annapolis Creed my first book. I love cooking, singing, and helping students become productive citizens.

Additional resources

My Websites:

annapoliscreed.com

mathpoop.com

alexalifeskills.com

pappyjordan.com

Acknowledgement

I would like to thank Carolyn Powers for her help in editing this book.

Annapolis Creed

A true story of about the resistance to racism at the United States Naval Academy and within the United States Marine Corps between 1972-1996. The is the story of the first African American to be named the Color Company Commander of the United States Naval Academy in June 1976. His selection starts a media frenzy because Midshipman Jordan B. Smith Jr. selected the first Color Girl (A Black Woman) breaking 155 years of Naval Tradition.